# Sex and Gender in the Pacific

This book examines sex, sexuality, gender and health in the Pacific with a focus on three key sets of issues: young people, culture and education; sexual and reproductive health and well-being; and belonging, connectedness and justice.

Bringing together the work of scholars from across the Pacific region, this innovative volume showcases traditional knowledge and diverse disciplinary scholarship of policy and practice relevance. In addition to focusing on relationships, health, education, family and community, chapters engage with a number of cross-cutting themes, including violence, justice and rights, and sexuality and gender diversity. Drawing on the diversity and richness of the Pacific, its cultures, languages and people, the book lays the foundations for future conversations and scholarship for, and by, those within the Pacific.

*Sex and Gender in the Pacific* is an important resource for students, researchers and practitioners working in Pacific studies, sexuality and gender studies, public health, nursing, public policy, sociology, education and anthropology.

**Angela Kelly-Hanku** is Senior Principal Research Fellow in the Sexual and Reproductive Health Unit, at the Papua New Guinea Institute of Medical Research and a Scientia associate professor in the Kirby Institute for Infection and Immunity in Society, Faculty of Medicine at UNSW Sydney, Australia. She has a background in the social sciences and public health and works at the intersection between culture, sexuality, gender, health and well-being. With colleagues, she has undertaken pioneering qualitative and participatory research in Papua New Guinea on a wide range of sexual, reproductive and maternal health issues. Angela is committed to working in a collaborative and empowering way with the communities she serves in her research, most notably young people, people living with HIV, people who sell and exchange sex, sexuality diverse men and transgender people.

**Peter Aggleton** has a background in the social sciences as applied to well-being, education and health. He holds senior professorial positions at a number of universities including The Australian National University in Canberra, UNSW Sydney, and UCL in London. He is an adjunct professor in the Australian Research Centre for Sex, Health and Society at La Trobe University in Melbourne. In addition to his academic work as a researcher, teacher, editor and writer, Peter has served as a senior adviser to UNAIDS, UNESCO, UNFPA and WHO. He has worked extensively across Africa, Asia and Latin America.

**Anne Malcolm** is a freelance consultant with a background in social work and public health. She has decades of experience working with global health programmes, providing specialist consultancy and support in programme management, design and evaluation to a range of government and non-governmental organisations, particularly in the Pacific region.

**Sexuality, Culture and Health series**

Edited by Peter Aggleton
*UNSW, Sydney, Australia*
Richard Parker
*Columbia University, New York, USA*
Sonia Corrêa
*ABIA, Rio de Janeiro, Brazil*
Gary Dowsett
*La Trobe University, Melbourne, Australia*
Shirley Lindenbaum
*City University of New York, USA*

This series of books offers cutting-edge analysis, current theoretical perspectives and up-to-the-minute ideas concerning the interface between sexuality, public health, human rights, culture and social development. It adopts a global and interdisciplinary perspective in which the needs of poorer countries are given equal status to those of richer nations. Books are written with a broad range of readers in mind, and will be invaluable to students, academics and those working in policy and practice. The series also aims to serve as a spur to practical action in an increasingly globalised world.

**Sex and Sexualities in Contemporary Indonesia: Sexual Politics, Health, Diversity and Representations**
Edited by Linda Rae Bennett and Sharyn Graham Davies

**Culture, Health and Sexuality: An Introduction**
Edited by Peter Aggleton, Richard Parker

**Gay Science: Intimate experiments with the problem of HIV**
Kane Race

**Young People and Sexual Citizenship**
Edited by Peter Aggleton, Rob Cover, Deana Leahy, Daniel Marshall and Mary Lou Rasmussen

**Sexualities, Transnationalism, and Globalization: New Perspectives**
Edited By Yanqiu Rachel Zhou, Christina Sinding and Donald Goellnicht

**Sex, Sexuality and Sexual Health in Southern Africa**
Edited by Deevia Bhana, Mary Crewe and Peter Aggleton

**Sex and Gender in the Pacific: Contemporary Perspectives on Sexuality, Gender and Health**
Edited by Angela Kelly-Hanku, Peter Aggleton and Anne Malcolm

For more information about the series, please visit: https://www.routledge.com/Sexuality-Culture-and-Health/book-series/SCH

# Sex and Gender in the Pacific

## Contemporary Perspectives on Sexuality, Gender and Health

**Edited by Angela Kelly-Hanku, Peter Aggleton and Anne Malcolm**

Routledge
Taylor & Francis Group
LONDON AND NEW YORK

First published 2023
by Routledge
4 Park Square, Milton Park, Abingdon, Oxon OX14 4RN

and by Routledge
605 Third Avenue, New York, NY 10158

*Routledge is an imprint of the Taylor & Francis Group, an informa business*



*British Library Cataloguing-in-Publication Data*
A catalogue record for this book is available from the British Library

ISBN: 978-0-367-69510-1 (hbk)
ISBN: 978-1-032-44263-1 (pbk)
ISBN: 978-1-003-14207-2 (ebk)

DOI: 10.4324/9781003142072

Typeset in Goudy
by MPS Limited, Dehradun

**For Arunai, Olawe, Nandame and Samenu, and all the children of the Pacific.**

# Contents

# Figures

# Table

# Boxes

# Contributors

**Herick Aeno** is a senior social researcher in the Sexual and Reproductive Health Unit at the Papua New Guinea Institute of Medical Research in Goroka, Papua New Guinea. His work explores socio-cultural and behavioural issues concerning sexual and reproductive health in Papua New Guinea. Within the Institute of Medical Research, he is currently coordinating a study on adolescent pregnancy.

**Peter Aggleton** has a background in the social sciences as applied to education and health. He holds senior professorial positions at The Australian National University in Canberra, UNSW Sydney, and UCL in London. In addition to his academic work as a researcher, teacher, editor and writer, Peter has served as a senior adviser to UNAIDS, UNESCO, UNFPA and WHO. The editor-in-chief of the journal *Culture, Health & Sexuality*, he has worked very extensively across Asia, Latin America and the Pacific.

**Jana Ali-Traill** is a mental health professional who has worked on the Fiji government's Child Help Line and in partnership with the Fiji Alliance for Future Generations and Emerging Leaders Forum Alumni. She is a counsellor and advocate who works mostly at grassroots level using social media to normalise conversations about sex, sexuality, gender and sexual reproductive health for all age groups in Fiji and the Pacific.

**Sophie Ase** was a senior researcher in the Sexual and Reproductive Health Unit at the Papua New Guinea Institute of Medical Research, where she worked for 10 years prior to her death in 2020. Her research included studies of sociocultural and biomedical understandings of cervical cancer and the acceptability of HPV vaccination, HIV prevention among key populations and the prevention of parent-to-child HIV transmission.

**Stephen Bell** Stephen Bell holds associate professorial positions in the Centre for Social Research in Health at UNSW Sydney, and the School of Public Health at The University of Queensland, Australia. He has published extensively on research pertaining to global health and social development, including the use of community-based, participatory and ethnographic research methodologies with excluded peoples in diverse settings in Africa, South-East Asia, Western Pacific and Europe. In addition to his academic work, Stephen has worked in research and strategy advisory roles with UNAIDS, UNFPA and WHO.

**Ruthy Boli-Neo** is a senior social researcher working in the Papua New Guinea Institute of Medical Research. She has been involved in implementing and coordinating social and public health projects in Papua New Guinea for more than 15 years, especially qualitative research focused on sexual and reproductive health including HIV/STI, gender and sexual diversity, human rights and gender-based violence.

**Karen Cheer** is a senior research fellow in the College of Medicine and Dentistry at James Cook University, Cairns, Australia. She has a diverse professional background with qualifications and experience in qualitative and cross-cultural research, library and information science, education and research administration. Karen's research focuses on social and cultural aspects of health and well-being in the Pacific region.

**Alec Ekeroma** is the Vice Chancellor of the National University of Samoa and holds an honorary professorship in obstetrics and gynaecology at the University of Otago, Aotearoa New Zealand.

**Dorothy Esau** is a Kwaio women's leader in Solomon Islands who works with local village community members to advance the health and well-being of women and girls. She facilitates and manages women's programmes with the Baru Conservation Alliance on Maliata and seeks to ensure there is a gender perspective in all the projects undertaken by the Alliance.

**David Taufui Mikato Fa'avae** is a senior research fellow at the University of Auckland, Aotearoa New Zealand. He is the grandson of Vika Lataheanga Fosita, Sione Taufui Mikato Fa'avae (paternal grandparents), and Melenaite Vetekina Jennings, Sione P. Tomasi (maternal grandparents). As a social scientist and education specialist, he has facilitated understanding of gender, intergenerationality and Indigenous masculinities in Aotearoa New Zealand and the Pacific region.

**Edmond S. Fehoko**, of Tongan descent, is a Health Research Council of New Zealand Pacific postdoctoral fellow in the School of Māori Studies and Pacific Studies at the University of Auckland, Aotearoa New Zealand. As a public health sociologist, Edmond's research interest is in mental health and addictions, cultural practices, education, public health, criminology and sociology.

**Katie Fitzpatrick** is an associate professor and Head of Te Kura o Te Marautanga me te Ako School of Curriculum and Pedagogy in the Faculty of Education and Social Work at the University of Auckland, Aotearoa New Zealand. Her research and teaching focus on health education, physical education, sexuality education, critical pedagogy, policy, poetic research methods and critical ethnography. She has led the writing of major national curriculum policy documents for the Ministry of Education.

**Debi Futter-Puati** is the Director of the Cook Islands campus of the University of the South Pacific. She is a social scientist and Indigenous health education specialist. Her research interests lie in investigating and promoting Pacific youth voice in relation to health and well-being issues such as sexuality, mental health including drugs education, Indigenous health and well-being, and the wider social determinants of health in Pacific settings. She is interested in Indigenous research methods and publishes within this space.

**Hilary Gorman** is a research fellow at Te Puna Vai Marama Cook Islands Centre for Research of the University of the South Pacific Cook Islands Campus and an independent consultant. She has extensive experience in research, evaluation, policy and development practice in the Pacific region. Her recent work has focused on gender inequality, sexual and reproductive health, and social policy.

**Relmah Baritama Harrington** is a Choiseul woman, midwife and nurse educator at the Pacific Adventist University, Atoifi Campus, Solomon Islands. She has worked as a nurse-midwife for more than 20 years, and has taught midwifery for 15 years. She is currently studying for a doctorate in health at James Cook University, Cairns, Australia where her research focuses on ways to improve family planning in Solomon Islands.

**Fiona Hukula** is a social anthropologist who specialises in gender in the Pacific and is currently Gender Specialist with the Pacific Islands Forum Secretariat, Suva, Fiji. Previously she was a senior research fellow at the National Research Institute in Port Moresby, Papua New Guinea where she undertook pioneering work on gender-based violence and sorcery related accusation related violence. Fiona remains an advocate against all forms of violence and works towards gender equity in the Pacific.

**Angela Kelly-Hanku** is senior principal research fellow in sexual and reproductive health at the Papua New Guinea Institute of Medical Research and a Scientia associate professor and Lead, Global Health Equity and Justice Group at the Kirby Institute for Infection and Immunity in Society at UNSW Sydney. She is a social scientist and public health specialist who has published extensively on matters pertaining to sexuality and gender, and sexual, reproductive and maternal health, in Papua New Guinea and elsewhere.

**Elissa C. Kennedy** is a medically-trained public health professional with 15 years' experience in adolescent health research and programming, focusing on sexual and reproductive health. She is Co-Programme Director of the Burnet Institute's maternal, child and adolescent health programme in Melbourne, Australia and Co-Head of global adolescent health, leading interdisciplinary research projects in the Pacific and East Asia.

**Tim Leach** is a former development practitioner who has spent many years working with human rights organisations in Papua New Guinea, principally the national association for people living with HIV, Igat Hope, and the Papua New Guinea organisation for men with diverse sexualities and transgender people, Kapul Champions. He has worked as a lawyer in HIV and public health, and human rights advocacy.

**Christine Linhart** is a senior lecturer in the School of Population Health, UNSW Sydney, Australia. She has extensive experience working in reproductive health in the Pacific region in research, policy and programme management. Her main area of focus over the past decade has been strengthening birth registration across the Pacific Island region, to ensure all children are able to exercise their right to a legal identity.

**Karen McMillan** is a former researcher with the School of Population Health at UNSW Sydney, Australia. She is a specialist in qualitative and ethnographic social research and has extensive experience working with hard-to-reach populations across the Pacific with a focus on sexuality and sexual practice.

**Elke Mitchell** is a senior research fellow in the UQ Poche Centre for Indigenous Health at the University of Queensland, Australia. She is a social researcher with expertise in qualitative, ethnographic and participatory research methods, and the evaluation of public health programmes. Her work focuses on the cultural and social aspects of sexual, reproductive and maternal health, HIV and other public health issues in Australia and the Pacific.

**Richard Nake Trumb** is an experienced social researcher in the Sexual and Reproductive Health Unit at the Papua New Guinea Institute of Medical Research. He has more than a decade's experience undertaking innovative research on issues such as masculinity, medical male circumcision for HIV prevention, the prevention of violence against women, TB control, pregnancy and young people, and people in HIV serodiscordant relationships.

**Jamee Newland** is a research fellow in the Global Health Equity and Justice Team at the Kirby Institute for Infection and Immunity in Society at UNSW Sydney, Australia. A social scientist with a cross-disciplinary background in public health, she has a strong interest in using participatory and arts-based research approaches to explore issues of sexual and reproductive health, gender and sexuality, infectious disease, harm reduction and disability across the Asia Pacific Region.

**Roannie Ng Shiu** is a Samoan Pacific health and human geography researcher. She is currently a director of the University of Auckland Centre for Pacific and Global Health, Aotearoa New Zealand. She was previously a researcher in the Department of Pacific Affairs at The Australian National University in Canberra.

**Riki Nofo'akifolau** is the Operations Lead of the Village Collective - a Pacific non-governmental organisation that works with schools to deliver culturally responsive relationship and sexuality education to Pacific youth in Aotearoa New Zealand. With expertise in health promotion, group facilitation and performing arts, Riki led the development of relationship and sexuality curriculum modules to enable teaching staff to better connect with Pacific young people, their families and local communities.

**Amanda Noovao Hill** is an associate professor at the Fiji National University. She is a clinical academic in the field of obstetrics and gynaecology and has a special interest in medical education.

**Priscilla Selon Ofi** is a social researcher in the Sexual and Reproductive Health Unit at the Papua New Guinea Institute of Medical Research. She is part of the research team undertaking a major study of adolescent pregnancy. Priscilla earlier worked on other studies of sexual and reproductive health, and is currently contributing to a study of the political prioritisation of STIs in pregnancy.

**Emmanuel Peni** is a human rights defender working with Project Sepik, a local non-governmental organisation providing support for leaders along the Sepik River in Papua New Guinea to resist exploitative and destructive economic developments in mining and logging. He is an author, a leader in promoting literature in Papua New Guinea, and a social entrepreneur. He is also the President of Kapul Champions, a national non-governmental organisation promoting the rights of men with diverse sexualities in Papua New Guinea.

**Asetoa Sam Pilisi** is a programme manager for the Knowledge Hub within the Office of the Associate Dean – Pacific of the Faculty of Medical and Health Sciences at the University of Auckland, Aotearoa New Zealand. He is also undertaking a doctoral study at the university with a focus on well-being amongst New Zealand born Pacific people. While a proud son of Central Auckland, Asetoa hails from the villages of Avatele and Alofi Tokelau (Niue) and Sato'alepai and Vailoa Palauli (Samoa).

**Manuel Rauchholz** is associate professor of anthropology and intercultural studies at Trinity International University, Illinois, USA, where he also directs the doctoral programme on intercultural studies. Since 2010, Manuel has developed and managed multiple research, educational and community development projects in Micronesia, where he was raised, and is involved in developing a community elementary school on the island of Tol. He has a long track record in publications in cultural anthropology on the study of kinship and exchange, migration, legal anthropology and topics such as human trafficking, sexual exploitation, human rights, economic development and the environment.

**Jioji Ravulo** is professor and chair of social work and policy studies at The University of Sydney, Australia. His father is iTaukei Fijian, and his late mother is Anglo-Australian. Such intersecting perspectives meaningfully inform his teaching, research and writing across the fields of mental health, alcohol and other drugs, youth development, marginality and decoloniality.

**Michelle Redman-MacLaren** is an Anglo-Celt Australian known for her ability to facilitate action-oriented research in a culturally respectful way in pursuit of positive health outcomes. Michelle is based at James Cook University, Cairns, Australia and with a social work background, facilitates participatory, decolonising public health research with peoples from the Pacific (predominantly Solomon Islands and Papua New Guinea) that is sensitive to culture, spirituality and gender.

**Kerry H. Robinson** is a professor of sociology, Director of the Diversity and Human Rights Research Centre, and member of the sexualities and genders research group in the School of Social Sciences at Western Sydney University, Australia. Kerry's expertise includes childhood, gender and sexuality; gender and sexuality diverse children; sexuality education; sexual citizenship; and gender and sexuality-based violence and harassment. Kerry currently has several research projects addressing gender in schools; the sexual harassment of LGBTQ young people in the workplace; and being trans in the early years.

**Rhonda M. Shaw** is an associate professor in sociology at Te Herenga Waka | Victoria University of Wellington, Aotearoa New Zealand. Her research interests include the sociology of morality and ethics, and empirical research on the donation and provision of human biological materials and services. Rhonda is a principal investigator on a Royal Society of New Zealand Marsden Fund project entitled Accessing Assisted Reproduction: Social Infertility and Family Formation.

**Telusa Tu'i'onetoa** is a Tongan doctoral candidate at The Australian National University, Canberra. Before beginning this work, she was a development practitioner for 16 years at the Australian High Commission in Tonga. She has extensive expertise in the design, implementation and review of development programmes.

**Errollyn Tungunaboe** is an obstetrician and gynaecologist based at Vila Central Hospital in Vanuatu.

**Meredith Tutumang** is a development practitioner and consultant with over 25 years of experience in leadership roles, specifically in the areas of health policy, business models, systems strengthening, governance, service delivery and government relations. More recently she was the Papua New Guinea Country Representative at the Burnet Institute, Melbourne, Australia.

**Lisa M. Vallely** is a senior research fellow at the Kirby Institute for Infection and Immunity in Society at UNSW Sydney, Australia and has a joint position at the Papua New Guinea Institute of Medical Research where she established a programme of research on maternal health. She has over 20 years' experience as a midwife and public health researcher working in low- and middle-income countries, most notably Papua New Guinea.

**Analosa Veukiso-Ulugia** is a Sāmoan academic in the Faculty of Education and Social Work, at the University of Auckland, Aotearoa New Zealand. She is committed to the empowerment of Pacific communities, specifically in sexual health and well-being. In 2020, she was awarded a Health Research Council of New Zealand Pacific postdoctoral fellowship to undertake a study of 'Nesian narratives – Enhancing sexuality education for Pacific communities,' which documents the development, piloting and evaluation of a Pacific resource toolkit on relationship and sexuality education for Pacific learners.

**Pinip Wapi** is a specialist medical officer, obstetrician and gynaecologist at Nonga General Hospital, Rabaul, Papua New Guinea. He is a clinician and teaches trainee health extension officers (resident health extension officers), resident medical officers, trainee midwives and undergraduate nursing students. He has a special interest in research.

**Stephanie Wheeler** is a field epidemiologist and registered nurse working to engage communities and frontline health workers in health security preparedness and response in Australia and the Pacific. Currently with the Ministry of Health and Medical Services in Solomon Islands to develop field epidemiology capacity, Stephanie thrives when working at the intersection between the scientific community and the real-world community.

**Alyce N. Wilson** is a public health physician and senior research fellow in the Maternal, Child and Adolescent Health Programme at the Burnet Institute, Melbourne, Australia. In addition to this role, she works as a senior medical advisor with the Victorian Department of Health and teaches science, medical and public health students at the University of Melbourne.

# Acknowledgements

We thank Sarah Hoile for her editorial assistance and support.

# 1 Introduction: Pacific values, practices and insights into sexuality, gender and health

*Angela Kelly-Hanku, Peter Aggleton and Anne Malcolm*

Some 30 years ago, reimagining the Pacific as an interconnected sea of islands rather than as a set of disparate lands and peoples, the Tongan scholar Epeli Hau'ofa (1994) offered an Oceanic way of understanding and viewing the great ocean, the islands and the people on the land, not as multiple but as one, in relationship with each other. In doing so, Hau'ofa offered an imagining of the Pacific from within, an imagining that was hopeful and empowering, acknowledging that the future of this sea of islands lay in the hands of the people of this great region – the single largest region in the world, connected by moana | ocean, and known for its geographical beauty, its diverse cultures, its many languages, its complex kin relationships, its exchange of culture and trade, its long history of voyaging and its commitment to protecting and nurturing the moana in harmony with the people.

There is no one agreed Pacific identity, and indeed there exist tensions concerning who and what might be included when it comes to thinking about the region. Geographically, for example, Papua New Guinea, and West Papua are frequently excluded from being in the Pacific, or at least separated out. In Aotearoa | New Zealand for example, the government announced in 2021 that it was considering re-classifying Fiji Indian people in the census data as Asians and not Pacific Islanders, a suggestion that caused major tensions within the diaspora in Aotearoa, with Fijian Indians insisting on being recognised as part of the Pacific (Rovoi 2021). Politically, Hawai'i, Palau, New Caledonia and French Polynesia (among other countries and territories) enjoy a complex status by virtue of being, respectively: a state of the United States of America, an independent country in free association with its former colonial ruler, a France *d'outre-mer* collectivity, and a France d'outre-mer *sui generis* collectivity. In each case, citizens may owe allegiance to both a colonial power (or not) and to one or more cultures of heritage.

Because of this, and the growing diaspora, there is much variation in how people identify, speak about themselves and how they identify with their cultural heritage (see, e.g., Ravulo et al. 2019; Burnett and Bond 2020) as well as where they live. Often used terms include Pacific, Pasifika, the Blue Pacific and Oceania. Others use Indigenous descriptors. These descriptors refer not only to

DOI: 10.4324/9781003142072-1

those whose lands and ways of life continue to be subjected to colonial rule, such as the First Nations people of Hawai'i and the Kanak people of New Caledonia, or the i-Taukei people who live alongside a large and influential population of Fiji Indians, but to all the people of Oceania. We recognise and support all the identities used by Pacific peoples in this book and see this diversity of identification as central to the richness of the accounts that follow.

The essays this book contains differ considerably from the images generated by outsiders, including colonisers, missionaries, European artists and researchers. These include portrayals of Pacific people as noble, seductive and exotic in the work of anthropologists such as Margaret Mead (1928, 1935) and Bronislaw Malinowski (1927), and in the paintings of Paul Gauguin and Henri Matisse. They also include stereotypical portrayals of Pacific people as uncivilised, savage, unknowable and warrior-like in the writing of Thomas Jefferson Jacobs (2014 [1844]) and Captain James Cook (1999). Together, these accounts and images create challenges for any proper understanding of the Pacific, its culture (s), its richness and diversity, and its peoples. They have been rightly challenged by many Pacific writers.[1] Contemporary understanding is made no easier by the tendency to divide the Pacific up into sub-regional configurations of Micronesia, Melanesia and Polynesia, using terminology steeped in the history of coloniality and the desire of Westerners to categorise Others (Tcherkézoff 2003). The importance of transcending these limiting and damaging tropes, and the need to think regionally, while treasuring diversity and heritage as contributors seek to do in this book, is reflected in the recent *2050 Strategy for the Blue Pacific Continent* (Pacific Islands Forum Secretariat 2022).

In the three decades since Hau'ofa first spoke of *oceanic people* in ways that were hopeful and empowering, there has been a rapid growth in thinking, feeling and writing about moana, in forms that are respectful of people's diverse ancestries and heritage.[2] This is particularly the case in respect of the importance given to traditional knowledge in guiding responses to the important issues of the day. Out of this work has come a painful reckoning with the role that colonisation (by Britain, France and other nations) and missionisation in the form of Christianity, have had on traditional knowledge systems, ways of living and ways of being. An example of this reckoning of Christianity with traditional Samoan knowledge and sexuality, for example, was provided by his Highness Afioga Tui Atua Tupua Tamasese Ta'isi Efi in an address given at the 2009 Parliament of the World's Religion. The subject later became the subject of an edited book (Suaalii-Sauni et al. 2014). In his address, Efi charts the impact that Samoan Christian sensibilities of guilt and sin had on ritual dances such as the *sa'ē*[3] and traditional marriage chants such as the *Salani tini* with phrases deemed too graphic now being omitted[4] (Efi 2014). Somewhat differently, it was recently evidenced in the Australian context where several Pacific players from a rugby league team refused on religious and cultural grounds to wear a PRIDE jersey with rainbow colours to indicate inclusivity (Ravulo 2022). Other colonising institutions too – such as universities and the 'academy' (Smith 1999), international agencies and non-governmental organisations – have been destructive of local practices and traditional ways of life and knowledge, much of it in the name of economic and social 'development' (Childs and Williams 2013). In consequence, there is growing acknowledgement of the tension that contact with Europeans (and others) has brought to Oceania.

Used throughout the region, plant fibres (often pandanus leaves) are chosen, beaten, often coloured, and woven together with skill and precision, creating stories and designs. Whether in Kiribati or Yap, in Vanuatu or Tuvalu, or in Bougainville or Hawai'i or any other part of the Pacific, mats are central to community life. They provide a place for people to come together, rest, connect, talk and resolve issues. Highlighting the cultural value of mats and their significance, one recent highly publicised example comes to mind. In 2021, the Aotearoa | New Zealand Prime Minister Jacinda Ardern gave an unreserved apology to members of the Pasifika community for what are now known as the 'Dawn Raids' (see, e.g., Anae 2012). Frequently arriving early in the morning at the homes of suspected overstayers, Police systematically and disproportionally targeted Pacific Islanders suspected of overstaying their visas/work permits. Many Pasifika people were deported and sent back to their homes of origin. The pain of these raids has been expressed in the arts as well as politics with the formation of the Polynesian Black Panthers (Anae 2012). As part of the much-awaited apology, and in respect of Pacific ways of dealing with conflict and wrongdoing, Ardern was covered in a mat of forgiveness by members of the Samoan community as part as an *ifoga*, a traditional Samoan ritual of apology.

Metaphors of weaving, focusing on conversation (not outcomes), taking the time to listen, being reflective and prioritising Pacific views and values, recur through this book, led by those for whom the Pacific matters most – Pacific islanders in the Pacific and in the growing diaspora elsewhere within the region. Pacific values and practices of communicating are evident in the contributions that follow, with every chapter referring to the importance of conversation and some specifically engaging directly with the practice of weaving and the importance of the mat. It is for this reason that we decided to include an image of a mat on the cover of this book, welcoming readers to sit with contributors as they listen to the stories authors have to share as they engage with matters of sex, sexuality, gender and health.

*Talanoa* is a word that can be found in several of the Austronesian language families spoken in the Pacific, most notably in Polynesia. A talonoa is a deliberate conversation that embodies cultural values of respect, flexibility, tolerance, fairness and openness (see, e.g., Robinson and Robinson 2005; Vaioleti 2006). It embodies a process that is circular and not teleological in that it starts with a specific endpoint in mind. Many of the chapters in this book refer to talanoa both as a process of knowing and learning, but also as a research method and a way of having a respectful conversation with others. We recognise that this volume itself is one such a conversation, it is not the be-all and end-all of what can be said about gender, sex and sexuality in the Pacific, or any other matter. We recognise too that its publication is void of the protocol and ceremony one would expect of a traditional talanoa. Despite this, we welcome and invite all readers from whatever seas, lands and seas of islands they come, to join a conversation with contributors who span the Pacific and include people living in, coming from, and with significant and enduring ties to Chuuk, Cook Islands, Fiji, Niue, Papua New Guinea, Samoa, Solomon Islands and Tonga.

## Pacific Scholarship and prioritising Pacific ways, views and scholars

We are writing at a very special point in time – with Pacific Scholarship increasing rapidly, and with growing priority given to hearing stories from and within, rather than 'of' the Pacific; the current work on climate change justice and securing the future of moana, and the people of the Pacific, is a case in point. New ways of working and of doing research within the Pacific have been and are continuing to be demanded. Some call this process one of decolonisation (Smith 1999), with Pacific Islanders moving from being the 'researched' to the researchers (see, e.g., Kelly-Hanku et al. 2021) in contexts where equitable partnerships are forged and guided from within the Pacific. This shift in scholarship, prioritising Pacific ways, views and scholars, is attributable to the leadership of those who have gone before, and those still working among us, with this book building on the important foundations laid by scholars and writers including, but certainly not limited to, Jemaima Tiatia, Maualaivao Albert Wendt, Epeli Hau'ofa, Fuimaono Karl Pulotu Endemann, Colin Tukuitonga, Teresia K. Teaiwa, Huanani-Kay Trask, Alec Ekeroma, Bernard Narokobi, Katerina Teaiwa, Karlo Mila and Val Kalei Kanuha. We thank them, and many others, for their insight and their work.

The essays within this volume add modestly to the growing body of scholarship *for and by* those within the Pacific, giving priority to new and emerging thought leaders and those whose work is important but often not heard about. In keeping with the respectful and emic perspective, we have sought to foster while developing this book, the vast majority of chapters are led by Pacific Island authors (of varying nationalities, heritages and identities), including activists and early career scholars as well as more established researchers. There are contributions too from Pacific people currently living in the growing diaspora, but regardless of current residence each and every chapter demonstrates a deep connection and commitment to the region, its diverse peoples, and the development of Pacific Scholarship.

## Book overview

The chapters included here have been carefully and respectfully crafted and woven together. They illustrate contemporary issues of sex, sexuality and gender and their implications for health, well-being, equity and belonging across this sea of islands. While the focus is sometimes on difficulties and problems, more generally the authors propose thoughtful, respectful and forward-looking ways of responding to these. Both individually and together, chapters showcase traditional knowledge and disciplinary scholarship that draws on interpretive, historical, developmental and legal traditions. The outcome is a robust and sensitive account of cultures, contexts and peoples.

Beyond appealing to those working in Pacific studies, gender and sexuality studies, health and development studies, and sexual and reproductive health and rights, the book will have relevance to students and researchers interested in gender, sex and sexuality in health, education, social work, psychology, sociology, anthropology and related disciplines. It examines issues of sex, sexuality, gender and health through a focus on three important, intersecting fields.

## Young people, culture and education

In this first section, authors detail meaningful and culturally respectful ways of including young people in research, policy-making and practice as active agents in their own lives. Chapters offer insights into youth-centred approaches to matters as diverse as gender-based violence and equality, sexuality and gender diversity, and developing and implementing culturally responsive relationships and sexuality education policy.

Education for young people presents specific challenges in relation to content and the way it is delivered. Jana Ali-Traill in her chapter 'Pacific youth-led sex positive responses and gender equity advocacy in Fiji' focuses on why engaging with young people and seeing them as key resources to address matters of gender equality, sexuality and violence is critical. She highlights how a focus on youth-led initiatives means engaging in new ways of creating connectedness and openness to discuss relationships. Her work highlights the pioneering use of social media to create a sex-positive youth culture in the Pacific as it connects the sea of islands to the rest of the world.

Analosa Veukiso-Ulugia and her co-authors in 'Weaving policy, theory and practice: Relationships and sexuality education and Pacific young people in Aotearoa New Zealand' discuss the history of Western-centric policy development in relationships and sexuality education and the process of restoring Māori voice and Pacific content in education policy in Aotearoa New Zealand. Weaving in Pacific concepts and values as part of relationships and sexuality education is to deliver a culturally responsive education to Pacific youth, reflecting the diversity of Pacific communities and the way in which these communities engage with each other and the broader environment.

In her chapter 'Inangaro | Desire: The 'writing in' of māpū | young Cook Islanders' sexual and relationship desires into resources for sexuality and relationships education' Debi Futter-Puati explores the experiences of young people in Kuki Airani | Cook Islands with regards to sex and sexuality education as part of the process of developing a culturally appropriate education resource. Using a Tivaevae framework that borrows from the traditional quilt-making process, the research explores the rich landscape of young people's experiences. The development of a sex-positive resource, based on the realities of young people, has been followed by its use in a range of educational settings with the aim of ensuring young people grow to become sexually healthy adults.

Jioji Ravulo in his chapter 'A Positive Youth Development approach to addressing sexual and gender diversity with Pasifika young people in Australia' proposes the use of this framework to support young Pasifika in their path to navigating and negotiating their evolving identities. Colonisation and Christianity have changed values and beliefs in relation to gender and sexuality and have introduced shame and stigma to practices and behaviour that were once understood and accepted within communities. The Positive Youth Development framework the chapter describes provides a safe and supportive space in which young people can explore and learn about the sociohistorical and sociocultural contexts in which sexuality and gender diversity may play out, and ways to affirm and feel value for their Pacific identity and heritage.

## Sexual and reproductive health and well-being

In this section, chapters move from offering a broad overview of sexual and reproductive health concerns to more specific issues of menstruation, infertility, pregnancy prevention and unplanned pregnancy. The chapters raise important issues about cultural and gender expectations, fear and shame, inter-generational communication and how access to services and technologies can improve the health and well-being of young people.

Alyce Wilson and her co-authors in 'Sexual and reproductive health needs, challenges and opportunities in the Pacific' provide an overview of these challenges and the socio-cultural determinants that underlie these. Limited health infrastructure, health worker shortages, the judgemental attitudes of some health workers and lack of confidentiality are some of the factors affecting women's access to health services. Cultural and customary practices, religious beliefs and gender inequality contribute to the poor sexual and reproductive health outcomes that women and girls too often experience. Wilson and her colleagues call for community-driven strategies to improve sexual and reproductive outcomes and the greater engagement of Pacific Islanders as researchers in the field.

Led by community leader Dorothy Esau and co-authors, 'Grassroots action for improved menstrual health of schoolgirls in East Kwaio, Solomon Islands' explores how a menstrual pad-making initiative, along with awareness-raising about menstrual hygiene and health, can transform health and educational opportunities for girls in rural settings. The authors highlight how a broader systems-based approach to working with families, communities and schools helped build a supportive environment in which the girls could interact without fear or shame and where they could feel empowered to continue their education during menstruation.

In 'From burdens to blessings: A Pacific perspective on infertility and assisted reproductive technologies in Aotearoa | New Zealand' Edmond Fehoko and Rhonda Shaw examine some of the barriers facing Pacific Islander women seeking treatment for infertility in Aotearoa | New Zealand. The authors used a talanoa to maximise openness in their discussions with women about the experiences they had had given the stigma associated with infertility. Family expectations, spiritual and cultural influences, and fertility treatment service concerns were key barriers identified in accessing assisted reproductive technologies. Finding safe ways for families to discuss sex and infertility, educating religious leaders and improving the cultural awareness of medical staff are identified as some of the ways to reduce these barriers.

In their chapter, 'Socio-structural influences on young men's experiences of sex, pregnancy and pregnancy prevention in Papua New Guinea,' Herick Aeno and co-authors provide important insights into the sexual lives of young men aged 15–19 years in a peri-urban and rural area in the Highland's region of Papua New Guinea and their everyday efforts to prevent pregnancy. In pursuit of knowledge about effective means of contraception and the resources to put into practice what they have learned, young men experience constrained sexual agency, but agency nevertheless, using the information available – however inaccurate, limited or misconceived – in ways to limit the likelihood of pregnancy. Their work reinforces the importance of listening carefully to what young people have to say and providing services that address their needs – in particular, their wish to pursue happy sexual lives, free from unwanted pregnancy.

Telusa Tu'i'onetoa and her co-authors in '*Fofola e fala kae talanoa 'a e kainga* (roll out the mat so that the family can talk): Unplanned pregnancy and support for young women and girls in Tonga' discuss the experiences of young women and girls who face an unplanned pregnancy in Tonga. Using the practice of talanoa, the authors explore attitudes to and knowledge about sexual and reproductive health, attitudes to contraception and the reactions of girls and young women and their families to unplanned pregnancy. Using a Tongan metaphor – Fofola e fala kae talanoa 'a e kainga – the chapter discusses the importance of gathering and talking to provide young women and girls with the opportunity to discuss concerns about sexual and reproductive health.

## Belonging, connectedness and justice

This final section of the book explores the role of custom, tradition and belonging to family and community as these relate to contemporary issues of gender and sexuality diversity, gender equity and violence, cultural identity in the diaspora, human rights and local justice.

Roannie Ng Shiu and co-authors in their chapter 'Moana masculinities in the diaspora: Cultural identity and performance on the dance stage and the sports field' examine the tropes of Pacific masculinity that characterise modern moana men and explore how they are enacted in male warrior dance performance and male sport. Colonisation and migration have resulted in many men living away from ancestral homes and losing contact with their cultural identity and community support. The authors discuss how involvement in dance performances can reconnect diasporic Niue men to their culture, strengthening their identity as Niue men. Similarly, while participation in Australian Rugby League has provided opportunities for many Pacific men to showcase their physical capabilities, doing so has also been instrumental to raising awareness about the broader inequalities Pacific men face while living outside their ancestral homes and reconnecting players to their cultural heritage.

Drawing on the rich history of material culture, Ruthy Boli-Neo and her co-authors in 'Making meaning out of objects: Self, connectedness and belonging among sexuality diverse men and transgender women in Papua New Guinea' discuss material objects of cultural and social significance to sexuality diverse and transgender women in Papua New Guinea. Everyday life objects such as booklets, jewellery, photographs and clothing are used to represent the social life of the owner. Through these objects, participants express an increased sense of self, belonging and acceptance. The narratives the chapter provides offer new insights into the lives of gender and sexuality minority Papua New Guineans who are frequently framed in public discourse as being at risk of sexually transmitted infections such as HIV and speaks to the importance of kinship and family, identity and self-courage, justice and human rights.

Written as a conversation, Emmanuel Peni and Tim Leach in their chapter 'Localising human rights for men of diverse sexuality, transgender women and people living with HIV in Papua New Guinea' focus in on human rights and how these are viewed from a Papuan New Guinean perspective. In their discussion, they explore dominant framings of human rights with respect to gender and sexuality diversity as well as people living with HIV. Their discussion focuses on how gender and sexual identity are understood locally and in doing so suggests that Western influences have contributed to increased discrimination and stigmatisation; human rights frameworks derived from Western discourses have further stigmatised people by labelling, naming and compartmentalising 'in order to give rights to people who already have them in communities.'

In his chapter on 'Family and gender violence in Chuuk, Micronesia' Manuel Rauchholz draws on long-term ethnographic research in Chuuk and with Chuukese people in the USA. He provides an overview of traditional family relationships and how their structure impacts how violence is positioned, made sense of and responded to. Driven by economic and social needs, Manuel looks at how changes to family and kin relationships and living arrangements in urban centres both in Chuuk and abroad exacerbate family and gender violence. Manuel concludes the chapter by highlighting the tensions young girls raised in the USA may face when returning home to their villages in Micronesia, having to learn how their bodies are gendered and sexualised in new and often very different ways.

We conclude this section with a chapter by Fiona Hukula titled 'Gender inequality and Pacific-led solutions for a global problem.' She begins by looking at data on gender inequality within the region with a focus on gender-based violence and women's representation in political leadership before providing an overview of political commitments and frameworks to tackle gender inequality. Fiona highlights the important role played by international development partners in providing the resources to enable action on gender inequality across the region. Without this support, existing frameworks and agreements remain unactionable. Using initiatives such as the Fiji Women's Crisis Centre and SafeNet as examples, Fiona highlights the importance of feminist organising, churches, actions led by men and boys, as well as creative visual methods in developing Pacific-led responses to gender-based violence.

When it comes to writing about gender, sex, sexuality and relationships in the Pacific, too often approaches in the past have been those of an outsider looking in (as exemplified in early anthropological, missionary and artistic work), as if there is something Other and exotic to be discovered. In editing this book, we have eschewed such an approach, preferring instead to insist that authors and those who figure in their chapters speak for themselves, and share their experiences from within the Pacific. Rather than dividing matters up socially, culturally or geographically, our goal has been to privilege the region and its relationship to itself, ensuring that throughout the story-telling Pacific voices remain central.[5] *Sex and Gender in the Pacific* offers a call for continued meaningful and respectful conversation that foregrounds Pacific values, practices and insights into sex, sexuality, gender and health. We hope you enjoy reading it, but most importantly that it serves as a resource for ongoing learning and conversation.

## Notes

1 For an examination of these and other Polynesian authors' contribution to the Pacific re-writing of colonial representations of Pacific bodies, see, for example, Keown (2005).

2 We refer to moana here both literally and figuratively but are conscious that this is also a generalisation, as third-generation Australian-born Winnie Siulolovao Dunn writes, referring to the stubborn Pacific muse, drawing on the work of O'Brien (2015); 'Not every Pacific Islander feels a connection to the ocean' (Siulolovao Dunn 2019). She pays particular attention to the members of the diaspora such as herself who were raised in Western Sydney, Australia, far removed from the ocean. Equally, we realise that some Islanders in the Pacific who live at altitude such as the Lelet people of New Ireland (Papua New Guinea), or the highlanders of New Guinea (West Papua, Indonesia and Papua New Guinea), may equally feel disconnected.

3 The sa'ē is a ritual dance in which the beauty and sexuality of the body could be shown and flaunted, with the lyrics of the songs meant to provoke a sexual response: Take your clothes off and throw them inside the house, And dance naked to the beat of the sa'ē. When the papaya is open to one side, Then you can tell which is sweetest (Efi 2014, p. 28).

4 Salani tini is a marriage chant that refers metaphorically to the sexual organs, yet there are lines considered too explicit and have been excluded from recent attempts to revive it. Such lines include 'Sacred sperm spew out' (Efi 2014, p. 29).

5 For an important, but historical set of examples, see Jetñil-Kijiner et al. (1970). For a recent example in the area of Pacific social work, see Ravulo et al. (2019). And for a forthcoming collection on environmental histories of the Pacific, see Beattie et al. (2022).

## References

Anae, M., 2012. All power to the people: Overstayers, dawn raids and the Polynesian Panthers. In: M. Sean, K. Māhina-Tuai, and D. Salesa (eds), *Tangata O Le Moana: New Zealand and the people of the Pacific*. Wellington: Te Papa Press.

Beattie, J., Jones, R.T., and Melillo, E.D. (eds), 2022. *Migrant ecologies: Environmental histories of the Pacific World*. Honolulu: University of Hawaii Press.

Burnett, R. and Bond, S., 2020. 'Pasifika' and 'I-Kiribati' identity in Aotearoa New Zealand: 'Dancing' and 'edge-walking' through multiple identities. *Asia Pacific Viewpoint*, 61 (2), 327–337. doi:10.1111/apv.12251

Childs, P. and Williams, P., 2013. *Introduction to post-colonial theory*. New York: Routledge.

Cook, J., 1999. *The journals of Captain Cook*. London: Penguin Classics.

Efi, Tui Atua Tupua Tamasese Ta'isi, 2014. Whispers and vanities in Samoan Indigenous religious culture. In: T.M. Suaalii-Sauni, et al. (eds), *Whispers and vanities: Samoan Indigenous knowledge and religion*. Wellington: Huia, 11–42.

Hau'ofa, E., 1994. Our sea of islands. *The Contemporary Pacific*, 6 (1), 148–161.

Jacobs, T.J., 2014 [1844]. *Scenes, incidents, and adventures in the Pacific Ocean: Or, the islands of the Australasian seas, during the cruise of the clipper Margaret Oakley under Capt. Benj. Morrell*. Charlestown: Nabu Press.

Jetñil-Kijiner, K., Kava, L., and Perez, C.S. (eds), 1970. *Indigenous Pacific Islander eco-literatures*. Honolulu: University of Hawaii Press.

Keown, M., 2005. *Postcolonial Pacific writing: Representations of the body*. London: Routledge.

Kelly-Hanku, A., et al., 2021. From the researched to the researcher: Decolonising research praxis in Papua New Guinea. In: S. Bell, P. Aggleton, and A. Gibson (eds), *Peer research in health and social development*. London: Routledge, 20–32.

Malinowski, B., 1927. *Sex and repression in a savage society*. London: Routledge & Kegan Paul.

Mead, M., 1928. *Coming of age in Samoa: A psychological study of primitive youth for western civilisation*. New York: William Morrow & Co.

Mead, M., 1935. *Sex and temperament: In three primitive societies*. New York: William Morrow & Co.

O'Brien, P., 2015. *Pacific muse: Exotic femininity and the colonial Pacific*. Seattle: University of Washington Press.

Pacific Islands Forum Secretariat, 2022. *2050 strategy for the Pacific Blue Continent*. Available from: https://www.forumsec.org/wp-content/uploads/2022/07/2050StrategyfinalWebV.pdf [Accessed 3 August 2022].

Ravulo, J., 2022. Don't blame Pacific Island cultures for queer fear. Blame colonisation. *Sydney Morning Herald* [online], 27 July. Available from: http://smh.com.au/sport/don-t-blame-pacific-island-cultures-for-queer-fear-blame-colonisation-20220727-p5b50c.html [Accessed 29 July 2022].

Ravulo, J., Mafile'o, T. and Yates, D.B. (eds), 2019. *Pacific social work: Navigating practice, policy and research*. London: Routledge.

Robinson, D. and Robinson, K., 2005. *"Pacific ways" of talk: Hui and talanoa*. NZ Trade Consortium Working Paper, no. 36. Wellington: New Zealand Institute of Economic Research (NZIER). Available from: https://www.econstor.eu/handle/10419/66100 [Accessed 15 June 2022].

Rovoi, C., 2021. NZ's Fijian-Indians want to be recognised as Pasifika, not Asians. *RNZ* [online], 1 April. Available from: www.rnz.co.nz./international/pacific-news/439637/nz-s-fijian-indians-want-to-be-recognised-as-pasifika-not-asians [Accessed 2 July 2022].

Siulolovao Dunn, W., 2019. Playing God with our lives and stories: The stubborn power of the Pacific muse. *Overland* [online], 2 April. Available from: https://overland.org.au/2019/04/playing-god-with-our-lives-and-stories-the-stubborn-power-of-the-pacific-muse/ [Accessed 29 June 2022].

Smith, L.T., 1999. *Decolonizing methodologies: Research and the Indigenous peoples*. Dunedin: University of Otago Press.

Suaalii-Sauni, T.M., et al., 2014. *Whispers and vanities: Samoan Indigenous knowledge and religion*. Wellington: Huia.

Tcherkézoff, S., 2003. A long and unfortunate voyage towards the 'invention' of the Melanesia/Polynesia distinction 1595-1832. Translated from French by Isabel Ollivier. *The Journal of Pacific History*, 38 (2), 175–196. doi:10.1080/0022334032000120521

Vaioleti, T.M., 2006. Talanoa research methodology: A developing position on Pacific research. *Waikato Journal of Education*, 12, 21–34.

Part I

# Young people, culture and education

# 2 Pacific youth-led sex-positive responses and gender equity advocacy in Fiji

*Jana Ali-Traill*

An uncomfortable silence filled the room. Curious eyes shifted from the packets of condoms on the table to each other, barks of nervous laughter broke the silence when I asked this group of parents and teenage children to share what the purpose of condoms was. No one said 'sex' or made eye contact with me. I was not surprised. Mixing parents and their older children together to discuss matters of sex is uncommon, especially in Fiji and the wider Pacific. Earlier on, local civil society organisations and non-profit organisations in Fiji identified that one of the contributing factors to poor sexual health outcomes among teenagers in Fiji was the lack of intergenerational communication about healthy and safe sex practices. This finding was further confirmed by a study conducted in Fiji on parents' perception regarding the delivery of sexual and reproductive health education in secondary schools (Ram et al. 2020). Discussing sex and sexuality is a culturally taboo subject. Young Pacific people are brought up to remain silent. Even if we want to speak out, or are asked to speak out, we fear being reprimanded by elders. To address this conversation gap, a counselling and sexual reproductive health and rights organisation based in Fiji held a series of intergenerational conversations in different communities to break the silence and help children and parents alike to talk about safe sex practices at home. While there were awkward moments and a reluctance to openly share, we opened the door for the beginning of a safe environment in which members of at least two generations could openly discuss and access accurate information about sex and relationships.

In this chapter, drawn from my own community activism and work in Fiji, I detail why a focus on young people and youth-led initiatives is important in the Pacific region. I illustrate this by examples of my counselling and advocacy work, the struggles encountered when trying to break down cultural and traditional barriers to address stigma and taboos around sex, sexuality and sexual and reproductive health, as well as mental health. I also discuss the use of social media as a way of connecting with my fellow Pacific Islanders to provide accurate and timely sex-positive information and advocate for gender equity in the region.

DOI: 10.4324/9781003142072-3

## Young people – The problem or a resource?

With half of the population in the region under the age of 23 years, the Pacific Islands are experiencing a 'youth bulge.' The youth bulge is the outcome of several factors such as the cultural norms of having a large family and hence high fertility rates and low uptake of and limited access to reproductive health services including contraception (Wilson 2020). This bulge – of which I am part – is often described as a problem, not a resource.

Despite the economic importance of young people to the societies in the Pacific, young people are not afforded the same emphasis, inclusion or space as elders to participate in formal and informal conversations and decision-making that affects us and our future. Young people are important influencers, we have skills and ideas to contribute to socio-economic stability, innovation, health and leadership. There has been some effort to redress this lack of inclusion in terms of climate change, with recent youth-centred initiatives regionally and in our island homes. Local initiatives by youth organisations, such as mangrove planting, tree planting and youth declarations, including one by 'Alliance For Future Generations,' a local youth organisation of which I am a part, are increasingly acknowledged in the local media (Turaga 2020). But more space needs to be given to ensure young people have a say in their future, especially as this relates to matters of sex, sexuality, gender and health.

Informed by my own professional experience and training in psychology, and as a Pacific feminist activist, I have come to realise that to actively engage young people in making decisions about their health, incentives need to be created by young people, for young people, with young people. Young people of the Pacific want to contribute, we have the ideas and the energy, we have also seen what happens when generations before us have remained silent. We want to move away from silently accepting this environment of shaming, denial and ignorance, openly embracing conversations, no matter how awkward the silences. We want to entwine our rich diverse Pacific cultures and traditions with our learning and lives as global citizens to develop safe spaces where every Pacific Islander, regardless of gender, sex, sexuality or age can live safely, be respected and speak/live their truth.

Our communities are still very traditional. Our leaders, parents and elders are shifting exceedingly slowly into a now more globalised world. Hierarchical structures act as a barrier to the inclusion of young people in discussion, minimising our role within our communities and the decision-making processes. There is so much that can be achieved if these hierarchical structures are reconsidered, allowing older and younger generations to form meaningful intergenerational relationships. By emphasising intergenerational connections, young people will be able to teach the older generations how to better connect to the outside world. This includes having an open mind and ability to understand how some revered cultural traditions hold us back, keeping us bound to cultures of violence, gender inequality and a negative mindset with respect to sexuality and sex. Learning to address the harmful aspects of our culture, and understanding that it is justifiable to make change, means that safer spaces can be provided for all Islanders.

There is a need to recognise young people in the Pacific are not just citizens of their island homes and the Pacific, but as global citizens, connected to young people elsewhere and exposed to their cultures and ideas. Young people – if their expertise is harnessed – are an asset to families and communities who can positively give back if we are given the tools and chances to be responsible and heard. Pacific youth are finding solidarity with each other and through this, grassroots-level youth-led interventions are flourishing in Fiji and elsewhere. We are pushing ourselves into conversations, creating spaces that allow us to become activists and advocates to help encourage other youths to become pro-socially engaged. We are a resource, not the problem.

## Efforts to address gender-based violence

Built on foundational values of love, care and community that emphasise the importance of family, the Pacific prides itself on upholding many diverse cultures and traditions. But it is these same cultures and religions that perpetuate the male-centred attitudes and patriarchy rooted deeply in its practices. Growing up in a society that often allows violence to continue without any consequences promotes the false idea that violence is intrinsic to Pacific lifestyles. Fiji has one of the highest rates of gender-based violence in the world (Rodriguez 2020). A UNFPA report suggests that 60%–80% of Pacific women are survivors of sexual and physical violence (UN Women 2014). Gender-diverse groups need to be part of the violence conversation in the Pacific as they are a vulnerable minority in communities that emphasise heteronormative lifestyles. Some societies in the Pacific are matrilineal (with land ownership being traced back through the matrilineal line) such as in Nauru, some parts of Fiji, Vanuatu, Solomon Islands, Papua New Guinea (including the Autonomous Region of Bougainville) and the Republic of Marshall Islands. However, the vast majority of Pacific societies are both patrilineal and patriarchal, men and the male line are given power in communities, over land, in places of worship, and at home, often placing women in vulnerable positions. Over the years there have been many efforts made by local and international agencies, such as Fiji Women's Right Movement, Wan Smol Bag, Oxfam and CARE International, Pacific Women Shaping Pacific Development, sometimes in partnership with government agencies, to resolve and bring to light the increasing incidence of violence across the Pacific.

As young Pacific people, we are repeatedly exposed to gender-based violence directly or indirectly, as both survivors and witnesses. Such violence has an everlasting impact on people's lives, it does not end when the perpetrator stops the abuse. It lives on among young girls who are more likely to become victims of gender-based violence and young boys who repeat the behaviour they have witnessed, sometimes becoming perpetrators (Pacific Women 2020). As children, we learn behavioural scripts from those around us, and often develop abusive relationships in and out of home if we ourselves have grown up with violence (Thomas 2020). Is this the legacy we wish to pass on to our children?

Addressing gender-based violence requires multidimensional approaches, at grass-roots and international levels. A common tactic used in the Pacific involves advocates going into communities to have open conversations with families in a language they understand about the causes and consequences of gender-based violence (Fiji Women's Crisis Centre n.d.). It is important that there is cultural fluency among those working in the area — understanding the sensitivity of cultural practices to allow for a better understanding of the causes of gender-based violence and why Pacific cultures retain the belief that women and gender-diverse groups' experiences, feelings and voices do not matter.

Not all sex is consensual. Sexual violence is an issue that has long affected the Pacific, with countries in the region recording levels of intimate partner physical and or sexual violence at a much higher rate than the global average of 1 in 3 women (World Health Organization 2021). Research shows that in Pacific Island countries such as Kiribati, Fiji and Solomon Islands, the lifetime experience of sexual and or physical violence by an intimate partner is two-thirds of Pacific women over the age of 15 (Asian Development Bank 2016).

Highlighting the intersectionality of Christianity and violence, a member of the Fijian Parliament uttered the following in late 2021: 'Sex offenders should be forgiven in the name of Christianity' (Nand 2021). This comment from a Fijian political leader serves to undermine all the work by feminist groups and survivor networks to bring perpetrators of violence to justice and hold them accountable under the law. The thinking that underpins these remarks places pressure on survivors to forgive, rather than the courts to hold perpetrators accountable.

The fear of being abused, shunned and shamed carries into these conversational spaces where many people will rather suffer in silence than speak out or seek information. Communities are often not open to advocacy against violence and gender issues, seeing it as an attempt to dissuade people from traditions and disciplinary practices. I have been in situations where traditional leaders argue there is no need for awareness, and that violence is not an issue. I have often wondered whether this is because they too have normalised violence in their homes or is it easier for them to just ignore what is happening in their communities?

Our people are shamed and silenced into a lifetime of violence. Violence is perpetuated by erroneous interpretations of our cultures and religions, enforced by those who benefit from enabling violence to vulnerable groups. But who has the right to speak on behalf of our Pacific cultures, and to continue to normalise these intergenerational curses and trauma? The devastating impact of the culture of silence, using shame and fear to convince survivors and witnesses that if they speak out, they are betraying their culture, religion and community. We need to work together to educate people that stopping violence and changing social norms is a shared responsibility.

Violence has no place in our Pacific culture. It is the result of a patriarchal society normalising the infliction of pain and placing it under the guise of cultural and religious norms to make it acceptable. Tackling violence should not be a solitary and silent battle; violence needs to be spoken about and addressed. Violence and abuse are everyone's business.

## The need for sex-positive education and counselling

Formal, skilled counselling as it is used elsewhere is itself still a relatively new concept in the Pacific, receiving increasing importance as it becomes an integral part of the response to cultures of violence as well as offering new models of interventions that emphasise the need for trauma-informed responses.

During my undergraduate psychology training, I had the opportunity to observe first-hand as a counsellor the mental health and sexual health inequities our society faces and how these contribute to the vulnerability of youth. The ability to openly talk about lived experiences with abuse, sexuality and sex lives is restricted by the beliefs and practices of traditionally patriarchal cultures and religious frameworks that are still widely part of the Pacific.

Sex-positive education and counselling aim to equip people with the knowledge and skills to understand and talk about their sex lives and their sexual and reproductive health rights. It celebrates sexual diversity and helps those of different genders and sexualities, those in polyamory or open relationships, and those in bondage, discipline, sadism and masochism and kink communities. In the Pacific, where heterosexual monogamous identities and relationships are hailed as the standard and 'right' way to be in love, to engage in sex, and to be married, it can be incredibly difficult for those who experience love, passion and pleasure in any way outside of the established standards to explore, discuss and celebrate such differences. Sex-positive counselling supports people to understand that it is okay and perfectly human to find love, happiness and pleasure outside of heterosexual monogamy. Sex-positive counselling is currently not offered in any of the counselling and/or psychology courses in universities across the Pacific. I had to take it upon myself to work one-to-one with established professionals in Fiji's human rights and sexual reproductive health and rights scene, to attend various workshops and seminars to familiarise myself with what sex positivity is and what healthy safer sex and sexual reproductive health rights are, and to learn about condoms and different types of birth control methods before I could combine this knowledge with that from my studies and experience as a counsellor.

Access to good quality sex-positive education would give myself and other young people in the Pacific the skills, knowledge and space and navigate a way into sex safely and healthily, to better make decisions, and address relationships more healthily and openly. As a counsellor, implementing sex-positive counselling in the Pacific allows me to bring clients to a better understanding and appreciation of themselves, where they are able to address issues and concerns in a holistic manner and ensure that there is cohesion between their physical, mental, emotional and sexual health.

'Maybe if she had made smarter choices, this would not have happened to her.' It was difficult to hear these words from a well-experienced counsellor, someone I had worked in partnership with on projects throughout my advocacy work. During a joint operation with other civil society organisations, we were discussing a transgender sex worker who had reached out for help after being raped by their client. This older counsellor stood by her statement, saying that as a woman of God she could not accept the lifestyle this woman lived and did not want to provide her with help, saying that what she needed was the Church. It is essential that there is more understanding and acceptance among counsellors about the lives of all Pacific Islanders, not just heteronormative, cisgender ones. As counsellors we need to ensure our judgements do not harm our clients, are not dismissive and/or do not further perpetuate stigma towards those whose gender identities or sexual practices are outside counsellors' experience or moral frameworks. Counsellors need to be trained and supported in this work, otherwise our judgements will prevent the very people we want to serve from seeking guidance, counselling and legal support.

The issues sex-positive counselling intends to address are more than just issues related to sex. Sex-positive counselling involves helping clients develop personal responsibility for sex and addressing internalised negativity and abuse. It also assists in normalising conversation between partners about stress and anxiety in relationships and sex, sexually transmitted infections, cultural expectations and differences in sexual stamina and desires.

Conventional counselling services have focused primarily on the survivor's physical and mental health traumas, with the intent of helping them find healthy coping mechanisms to live their everyday lives, creating a long-term plan that helps them address traumas, maintain a healthy lifestyle and mental health. Very rarely is there conversation about the detrimental impacts that sexual violence can have on a person's sex life and a survivor's ability (let alone their desire) to re-engage in healthy, meaningful and pleasurable sexual relations. 'I want to have sex again!' shared by a client of mine who was a survivor of sexual assault. She had received counselling to help cope with trauma from her assault and to cope with daily life. But no one had considered helping her reintegrate back into a safe and healthy sex life, something she desired.

Across the Pacific, routine counselling rarely considers how to rebuild the survivors' connection with sex and relationships. But with such high rates of sexual assault and rape in our region, we need to more actively help those who want to re-engage and safely navigate their way back into intimacy, relationships and sex. Sex-positive counselling does not make one's sexuality or sex life the sole focus of the treatment, it allows clients to explore their sexuality and their sex lives, connecting these with their daily lives in a non-judgemental beneficial method.

The woman I counselled thought about sex often and wanted to re-engage in sex, to be intimate with someone and be able to feel pleasure from an act she once enjoyed, but struggled with the idea that the pleasure and joy she enjoyed with sex was no longer hers to enjoy. She had been raped in her family home by her uncle, a man she had lived with for her entire life. He justified his actions as, 'wanting to teach her a lesson,' and that this would not have happened to her if she had remained chaste until marriage. Her uncle took her sexual liberation as an attack on the family and their values. The woman's relationship with sex had been damaged. The trauma and guilt she felt placed her in an unsure place, wondering if she did deserve what her uncle did to her and whether if she had just followed the societal pressure of being a quiet chaste woman, this would never have happened. Discussions of daily coping, what sex meant to her, and her outlook and expectations towards sex and relationships were explored with psychological, physical and social health aspects, allowing her to breakdown her sexual well-being into components to identify the parts that needed to be addressed. The sex-positive counselling sessions helped her rebuild her relationship with sex in a protected environment showing compassion, not condemnation.

I have taken part in several sexual and reproductive health and rights focused community awareness programmes, where we would often hand out free condoms with demonstrations on how to use them. During one of these events, there was a group of friends, young people aged 18 or so, who took an interest in the condom demonstration. I took the chance to ask the group what they knew about condoms. The youths explained that in their *yasa* (neighbourhood), it was common practice for people to use small plastic bags and ice-block wrappers as makeshift condoms. Lack of access to condoms and understanding their importance in safer sex and sexual hygiene has led to generations of youth constantly putting ourselves at risk. After a discussion with my colleagues, we discovered that using makeshift condoms was a common practice throughout Fiji. Given these widespread experiences, it is important that sex positivity is reinforced in counselling and educational spaces, alongside the need for reliable access to condoms, possibly through youth-led groups to help ease the fear of accessing these services elsewhere.

Sex-positive education and counselling offer understanding, validation and healing by exploring and bringing awareness to all facets of the client's situation. To be able to use such an approach in the Pacific, culturally relevant knowledge is needed to address sexual health, sexual hygiene, sexual trauma, sexual violence, and gender and sexuality diversity. Using a sex-positive framework in counselling and education allows people to become more consciously aware of how culture and religion have created negative social attitudes towards sexuality, allowing them to navigate a balanced relationship with their sexual lives, values and beliefs.

## Youth-led digital initiatives – For youth, by youth

Coconut wireless, a term used in the Pacific referring to how quickly news travels by word of mouth, had spread it that I worked for a non-governmental organisation, that I was very open to discussing and helping people in talking about mental health, trauma, sexual and reproductive health and rights, and matters of sex. Soon enough, I was being contacted by people from all over Fiji and from other Pacific Island countries for information. I realised how devoid of opportunities and spaces the Pacific is when it comes to learning about sexual and reproductive health and rights safely in the context of our Pacific cultures. I decided to use my social media platforms, something that connects others with me, as a way of sharing experiences and knowledge, and hopefully encouraging other young people to seek help from established services as needed. I began by creating infographics of the different services available and ways to handle mental health and sexual health (see Figure 2.1). I worked with the Vosa

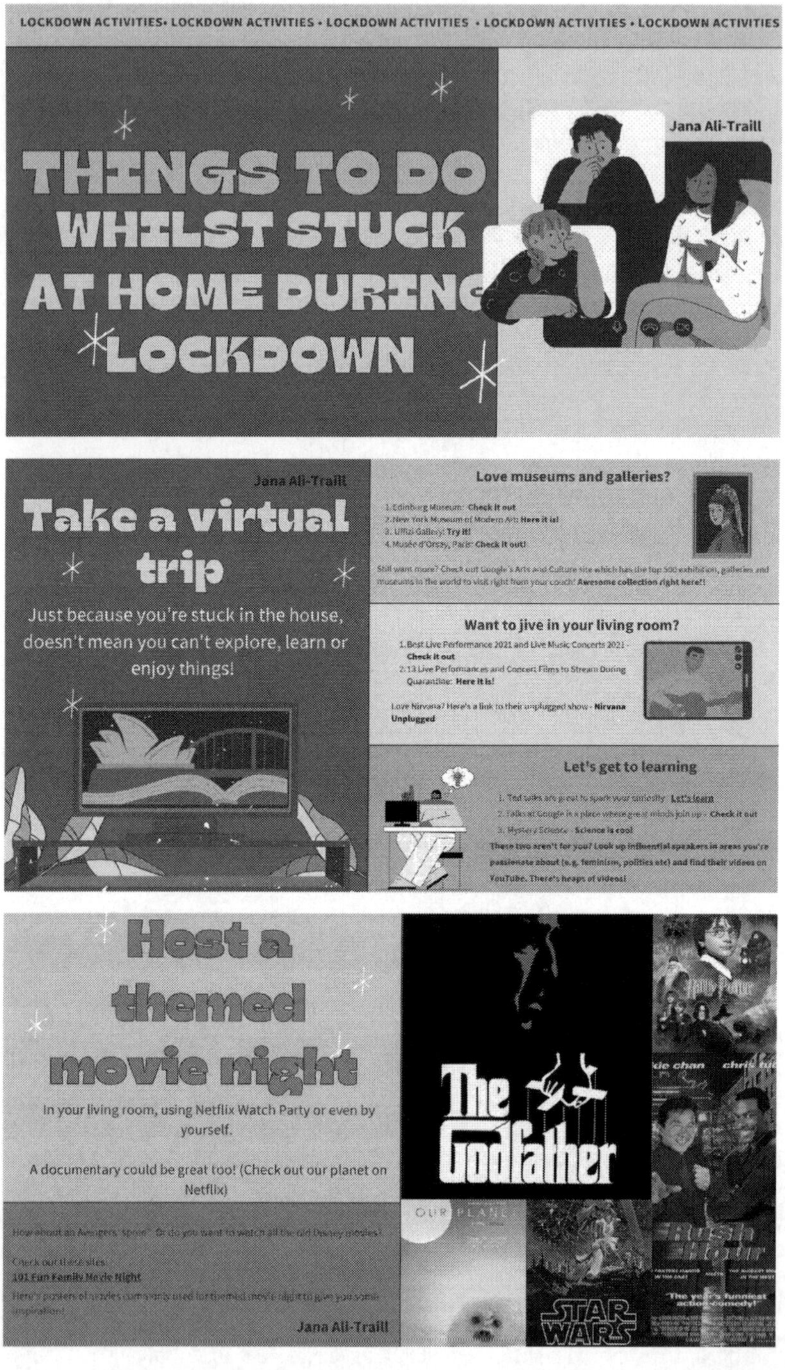


*Figure 2.1* Advertisements for podcast and webinars.

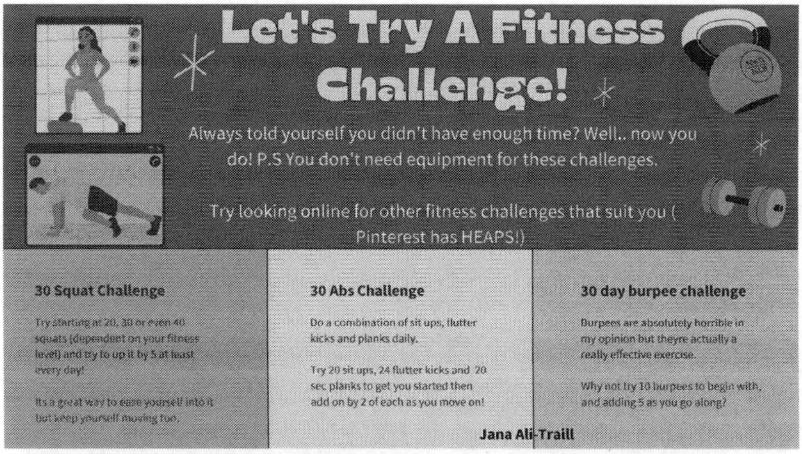


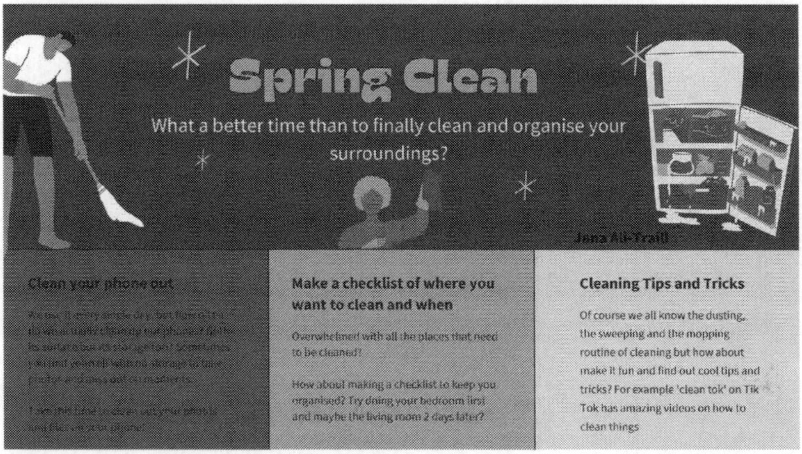


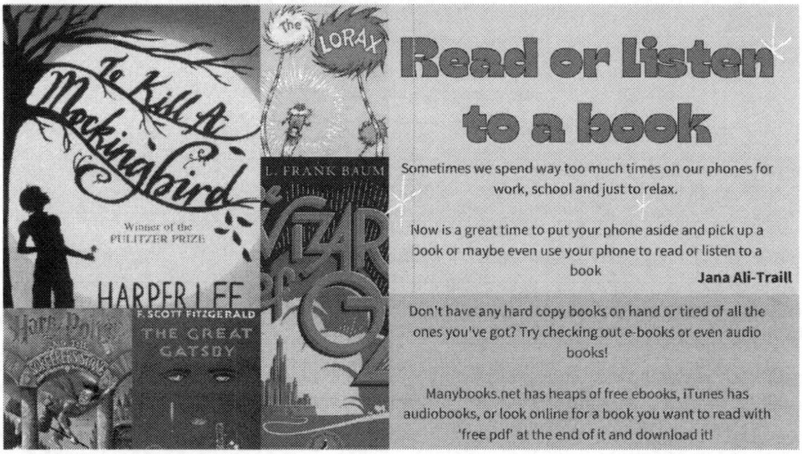


*Figure 2.1* (*continued*)

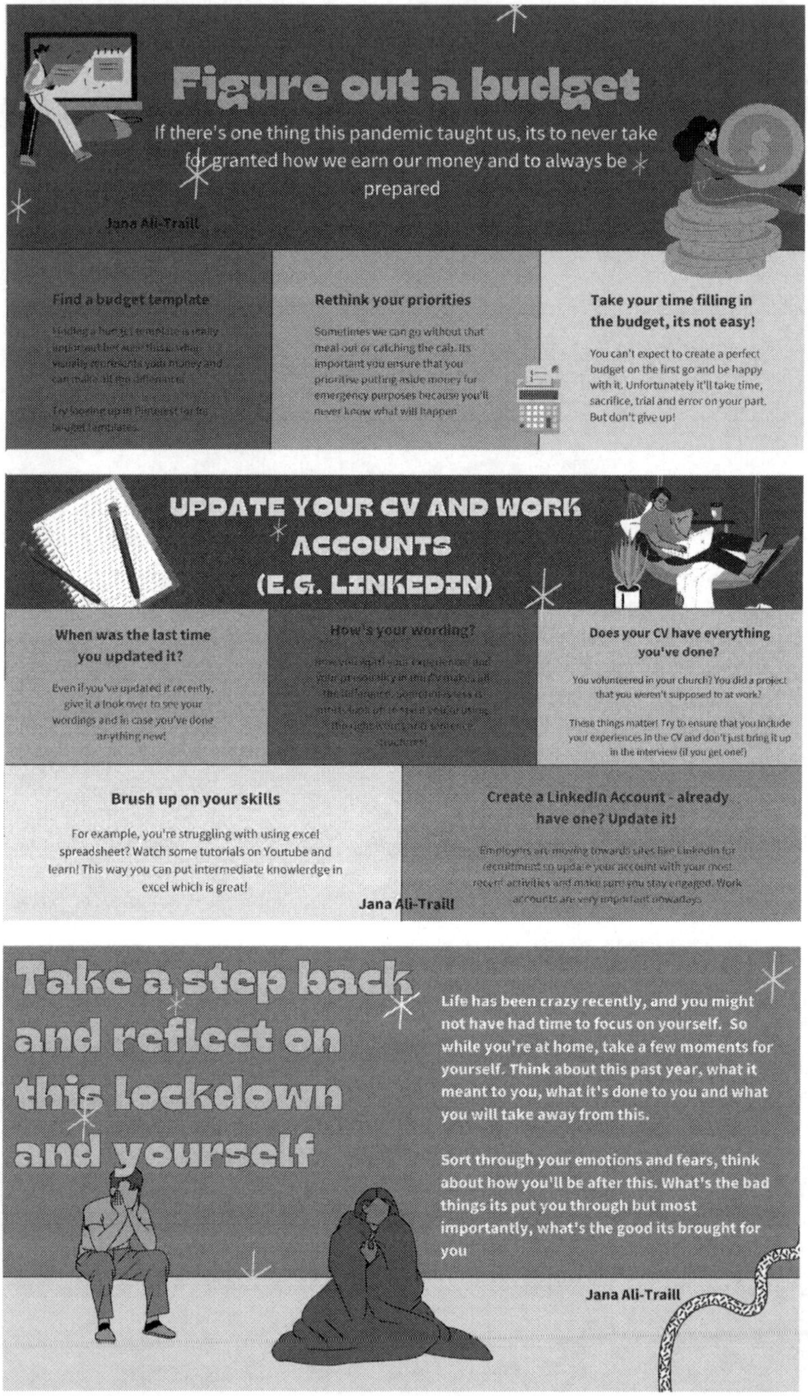


*Figure 2.1* (*continued*)

Podcast team (supported by the World Bank in the Pacific and Papua New Guinea) on the topic of Sex and Relationships in the Pacific.[1] Acknowledging the power of social media and the importance of grassroot initiatives in reaching other Pacific youth, I have worked with well-known Fiji activists and advocates to host numerous 'Twitter Spaces' via a feature that allows people to connect on a voice call on Twitter. This facilitated two-way informal but educational conversations with people on topics of mental health and sex.

Young people are connected to each other using new technologies that rely on online digital spaces in ways no other generation has; digital spaces have become an intrinsic part of life. We are often described as 'digital youth' (Erstad 2012, p. 25). Our transition into adulthood has been influenced by these new technologies and its tools. The emergence of new technology has affected the way Pacific Islanders access information, helping us develop new attitudes with sex and relationships.

When parents and or guiding elders (community leaders, church leaders, teachers etc.) spread non-sex positive messages focused solely on pregnancy and STI risks without elaborating on love, feelings, relationships, sexual impulses and desires, dissatisfied youth will turn to other sources to fill the information gaps, regardless of whether this information is provided by reliable or unreliable sources. One study found that whilst peers still play an important role in providing information or misinformation about sex, digital spaces are the most frequently used sources of relationship, sexual and reproductive health information for young people (Livingstone and Mason 2015, p. 23). Such spaces provide opportunities to quickly, easily and anonymously access information without fear of being ridiculed or admonished about sexuality, sex, menstruation, safety, gender and sexuality, relationships and our bodies.

Digital youth initiatives are part of a new movement that sees youth advocates and organisations guiding and supporting young people to use digital media and digital spaces to acquire useful knowledge and skills (social, educational, personal and sexual).

The art of storytelling is an integral part of Pacific cultures, it is how we have passed on stories and information through the generations, contributing to our *mana* (spiritual power and/or force) and our history. It is how we have learned from our elders, and how one day we will teach the children of our generation. Podcasts, as a form of audio entertainment that allows people to download and stream audio recordings, are a great way to share information with listeners, involving a *talanoa* (meaningful conversation) to share ideas, teach skills and to gather information. Whilst podcasts do not involve live interaction, they do allow people to listen to and learn away from stigma and shame, within a safe, comfortable, even secret, space if needed. Podcasts bridge the gap from our familiar Pacific cultural storytelling with the use of technology.

Webinars are another digital space used by youth advocates and organisations to disseminate sex-positive education information. I have found that in webinars, there is a lot more teaching than interaction than in other digital spaces. In the webinars that I have contributed to, we created our own questions to ask that would hopefully encourage attendees to ask questions or spark more conversation. Following these webinars young people have reached out after the sessions saying things such as 'I did not want anyone to hear my question, could you please explain this further?' or 'People I know were in the Zoom call, and I did not want them to tell my family I was asking questions.' Even if we, as civil society and non-profit organisations, do our best to create a safe environment for discussion, there will always be fear of a breach of privacy and trust when it comes to taboo subjects, especially in group settings.

Having recognised that social media platforms are an integral part of the lives of young people, the many Pacific civil society and non-profit organisations have created social media accounts to allow youth to access information about their services privately and easily, with some even allowing users to receive counselling through direct messaging. Advocates have started to use our own social media accounts as drivers of information by creating content (e.g., videos, infographics, text) that is easily shareable.

Digital spaces are continuously evolving with numerous platforms and a rich diversity of information being made available, creating opportunities for young people to access, share and create new knowledge. Digital youth initiatives are developing here in the Pacific, growing a 'for youth by youth' educational initiative. This offers young people the possibility to access and interact with sexuality education in a safe and non-judgemental environment that is often not offered in homes, communities or schools.

## Conclusion

Young people are a powerful collective force of change, we can be the spearheads of social transformation using our exposure to the globalised world and flow of information through digital spaces, and bringing this new way of living home to unite it with our Pacific beliefs. To advance sexual and reproductive health and rights, youth need to be heard in every space, especially where the decisions made by leaders are going to affect young people both today and in the future. It is the youth who are going to break intergenerational traumas and cycles.

In too many of our communities, sex and sexuality remain taboo subjects, gender-based violence is normalised, and fear runs rampant. Without any interventions, we as Pacific youth carry these teachings with us and then in turn we teach our young ones, allowing intergenerational cycles of abuse and trauma to repeat indefinitely. Without any guidance and safe space in which to talk about these issues, uninformed and inexperienced youth often turn to each other or to the Internet for help. Sometimes this can prove to be more harmful than helpful with the lack of appropriate guidance to guide young people to the correct and safe information.

We are not being prepared for the world that we will one day lead. Every young person has the right to be properly educated and informed about their physical, mental and sexual health in a setting that is safe and free from stigma. This right also extends to being able to access services that address these areas.

We need to educate and empower ourselves to understand the rights we have to safely access services, and how to use digital spaces to empower ourselves and others with knowledge.

We, the young people of the Pacific are the legacy of our ancestors who crossed oceans and toiled the lands, we are the sons and daughters of our families who survived hardships and kept the islands going as the world passed us by. We, the Pacific Youth, are the ones who are taking our island homes into the future with our *mana*, with connections to the globalised world, and with our education, carrying our legacy and developing spaces in the homes our ancestors built for us.

## Note

1 Link to the podcast: https://omny.fm/shows/vosa/vosa-season-2-episode-2-navigating-sex-and-relatio

## References

Asian Development Bank, 2016. *Gender statistics: The Pacific and Timor-Leste.* Mandaluyong, Philippines: Asian Development Bank. Available from: https://www.adb.org/sites/default/files/publication/181270/gender-statistics-pacific-tim.pdf [Accessed 26 January 2022].

Erstad, O., 2012. The learning lives of digital youth – Beyond the formal and informal. *Oxford Review of Education*, 38 (1), 25–43. doi:10.1080/03054985.2011.577940

Fiji Women's Crisis Centre, n.d. 5th regional meeting: Culture, religion still barriers in work to eliminate gender-based violence. *Fiji Women's Crisis Centre* [online]. Available from: http://www.fijiwomen.com/research/research-archive/5th-regional-meeting-culture-religion-still-barriers-in-work-to-eliminate-gender-based-violence/ [Accessed 26 January 2022].

Livingstone, S. and Mason, J., 2015. *Sexual rights and sexual risks among youth online: A review of existing knowledge regarding children and young people's developing sexuality in relation to new media environments.* London: European NGO Alliance for Child Safety Online. Available from: https://archive.crin.org/sites/default/files/sexual_rights_and_sexual_risks_among_youth_online.pdf [Accessed 26 January 2022].

Nand, E., 2021. Womens' rights group calls out Bulanauca. *FBC News* [online], 22 Sept. Available from: https://www.fbcnews.com.fj/news/parliament/womens-rights-group-condemns-bulanauca/ [Accessed 26 January 2022].

Pacific Women, 2020. Ending violence against women. *Pacific Women* [online]. Available from: https://pacificwomen.org/our-work/focus-areas/ending-violence-against-women/ [Accessed 2 September 2021].

Ram, S., Andajani, S., and Mohammadnezhad, M., 2020. Parent's perception regarding the delivery of sexual and reproductive health (SRH) education in secondary schools in Fiji: A qualitative study. *Journal of Environmental and Public Health*, 2020, 3675684. doi:10.1155/2020/3675684

Rodriguez, L., 2020. This small nation has one of the highest rates of gender-based violence in the world. *Global Citizen* [online], 15 September. Available from: https://www.globalcitizen.org/en/content/fiji-introduces-gender-based-violence-plan/ [Accessed 26 January 2022].

Thomas, E., 2020. How data is improving justice for gender-based violence in Fiji. *Open Global Rights* [online]. Available from: https://www.openglobalrights.org/data-improving-justice-gender-based-violence-fiji/ [Accessed 26 January 2022].

Turaga, S., 2020. Online training on backyard gardening being done by Alliance for Future Generations Fiji. *Fijivillage* [online], 1 May. Available from: https://www.fijivillage.com/news/-xf54r8/?fbclid=IwAR2RDEmGRHSybKbU8WnPY6GoYJPxtAtRTMoJRdr6xWFKk-iSZqB5wAh0M4bw#.XquBGtyOocY.facebook [Accessed 26 January 2022].

UN Women, 2014. *Climate change disasters and gender based violence in the Pacific*. Suva: UN Women. Available from: https://asiapacific.unwomen.org/en/digital-library/publications/2015/1/climate-change-disasters-and-gender-based-violence-in-the-pacific [Accessed 26 January 2022].

World Health Organization [WHO], 2021. Violence against women. *World Health Organization* [online], 9 March. Available from: https://www.who.int/en/news-room/fact-sheets/detail/violence-against-women [Accessed 26 January 2022].

Wilson, C., 2020. Demanding the future: Navigating the Pacific's youth bulge. *Lowy Institute* [online], 8 July. Available from: https://www.lowyinstitute.org/publications/demanding-future-navigating-pacific-youth-bulge#sec42956 [Accessed 26 January 2022].

# 3 Weaving policy, theory and practice: Relationships and sexuality education and Pacific young people in Aotearoa-New Zealand

*Analosa Veukiso-Ulugia, Riki Nofo'akifolau and Katie Fitzpatrick*

## Introduction

In September 2020, the New Zealand Ministry of Education (MOE) released updated curriculum policy guides for relationships and sexuality education in all state primary and secondary schools in Aotearoa-New Zealand (Aotearoa-NZ). Addressing students in years 1–8 (ages 5–12) and years 9–13 (ages 13–18), these policy documents aim to structure curriculum practice in relationships and sexuality education for all schools (MOE 2020a, 2020b). The policies take account of, and are inclusive of, diverse Pacific islander communities in Aotearoa-NZ. Significantly, they include models and content that emerge from, and speak to, Pacific cultures and knowledge systems in Aotearoa-NZ.

In this chapter, we[1] reflect on the inclusion of Pacific content and how this disrupts a long history of Western-centric policy development in the area of relationships and sexuality education, in one setting in the region. In addition, this inclusion creates productive tensions, as different knowledge systems appear alongside one another and interact in official state-sanctioned and national education policies. We also explore how engaging Pacific concepts is not only a matter of content and outcome, but also, importantly, one of process.

We begin by discussing issues of ongoing colonisation in policy-making and the efforts to restore and privilege the voices of Indigenous Māori. We then explore the cultural practices and knowledge systems that inform the inclusion of Pacific content in these relationships and sexuality education policies. We conclude with narratives of relationships and sexuality education in practice with Pacific communities in Aotearoa-NZ and offer some reflections about the possibilities that such policy moves can enable for those committed to relationships and sexuality education practice in ways that value and respect Pacific cultures and approaches to learning, sexuality and relationships.

DOI: 10.4324/9781003142072-4

## Policy-making

Official government policy documents such as the relationship and sexuality education policy guides, set directions for practice. These documents are often aspirational, and represent the complexity of politics in articulation with social and historical contexts. Mundy et al. (2016, p. 8) note that

> [t]here is an important distinction between policies as meta-discourses that shape what can be thought (policyscapes); policies as formalized rules and regulations; and policies as socially constructed enactments that span text and practice. Policy involves all three layers of action, including processes both before and after text production, and sometimes including formal evaluation processes.

The policies under discussion here are a product of these 'policyscapes,' which frame what is possible in any given social and historical period. In that sense, our reflection here offers a response to contemporary wider social concerns and health research, as well as to other state-sector policy moves. Education policy documents inevitably emerge at the intersection of tensions between global policy levers, localised concerns and cultural histories. Ball et al. (2012, p. 6) note that 'We see policy enactments as a dynamic and non-linear aspect of the whole complex that makes up the policy process, of which policy in school is just one part.'

In a sense, therefore, current relationships and sexuality education policies are an expression of a wider network of research, activism and practice. Importantly, current policies do not precede practice but, rather, interact with practice and wider social contexts in complex ways. For instance, relationships and sexuality education policies can be seen as reflecting political agendas around health and well-being, articulating what is currently occurring in schools, and imagining what is possible in Aotearoa-NZ. Such policies project future possibilities and express past practices and discourses. In this sense, policies – even as written documents – are not static but rather shifting and changing, echoing past and future relationships and sexuality education discourse. New policy must be read in relation to the ongoing impacts of colonisation in Aotearoa-NZ. Policy documents tend to reproduce rather than challenge colonial power relations. Deeply embedded in this is a history of embedded structural and epistemological racism that privileges white cultures, values and norms over others. Linda Tuhiwai Smith (1999, p. 65), explains that in education, epistemological racism works to hierarchise knowledge:

> Academic knowledges are organised around the idea of disciplines and fields of knowledge. These are deeply implicated in each other and share genealogical foundations in various classical and Enlightenment philosophies. Most of the 'traditional' disciplines are grounded in cultural world-views which are either antagonistic to other belief systems or have no methodology for dealing with other knowledge systems.

Earlier versions of these relationship and sexuality education policies were largely framed by Western approaches. In Western nation-states, these typically reflect individualistic, medicalised, liberal and secular approaches to sex (see Allen and Rasmussen 2016). While Indigenous, Pacific and other non-Western concepts are not entirely absent from previous policy articulations in Aotearoa-NZ, these worldviews are not centralised. The revised policies contain dedicated spaces for Pacific concepts and perspectives, and they give school communities specific advice on engaging with Pacific students and their families.

Recent research in Aotearoa-NZ shows that children and young people are increasingly questioning gender and sexuality binaries but that many schools are struggling to respond, or worse, are considered unsafe spaces for young people who identify in non-binary ways or as gender, sex and sexuality diverse (see Clark et al. 2014; Fenaughty et al. 2021). In Aotearoa-NZ, sexuality education in state schools tends towards exclusively secular content; whereas state-integrated[2] schools offer religious and faith-based approaches to relationships and sexuality. Content in many state schools privileges heteronormative binary identities, as well as centres upon Western-centric and secular notions of gender and relationships. This directly contrasts with many Pacific cultures that recognise non-binary approaches to gender. For example, *fa'afafine* (Samoa) and *fakaleitī* (Tonga) are terms that refer to people who are physically male but who are said to 'have the spirits of women' or 'behave in the fashion of a woman' (Pulotu-Endemann and Peteru 2001). The acronym MVPFAFF appears in the glossary of the revised relationships and sexuality education policies in order to acknowledge these Pasifika diverse gender identities or expressions, and reference is made to *māhū* (Hawaii and Tahiti), *vaka sa lewa lewa* (Fiji), *palopa* (Papua New Guinea), fa'afafine (Samoa), *akava'ine* (Cook Islands), fakaleitī or *leitī* (Tonga) and *fakafifine* (Niue) (Farran 2010; MOE 2020a, 2020b). These identities and expressions are unique to Pacific cultures and do not fit neatly into Western categories of gender and sexuality identity.

The intertwining nature of culture and religion, primarily the influence of Christianity amongst many Pacific communities, is also important when exploring policy initiatives and practice (Veukiso-Ulugia 2012; MOH 2020). Current relationships and sexuality education efforts in Aotearoa-NZ tend to be informed by secular understandings and values, and yet faith and spiritual beliefs are an important element of well-being for Pacific communities (MOE 2018; MOH 2020). Given these complex intersections, how can national policies for state schools engage such variation and diversity?

## Pacific concepts in (health) policy

Given Pacific peoples' unique relationship with Māori, efforts to weave Pacific frameworks into Aotearoa-NZ policy may be viewed as a responsive policy approach in formulating responsive policy. Māori, the *tangata whenua* (Indigenous people) of Aotearoa-NZ, share a special relationship and history with Pacific communities, long preceding Western contact. While the terms 'Pacific peoples' or 'Pasifika' are often used to describe the diverse cultures of peoples from Polynesia, Melanesia and Micronesia, in the Aotearoa-NZ context, they commonly refer to people from Polynesia, namely Sāmoa, Tonga, the Cook Islands, Niue, Tokelau and Tuvalu, and from Melanesia, usually only Fiji.

Pacific peoples currently comprise 8.1% of the total population; approximately half of this group are of Sāmoan descent, followed by Tongan and Cook Islands Māori (Statistics New Zealand 2019). While Pacific peoples are the fourth-largest ethnic group, behind European and Asian, almost two-thirds of Pacific people were born in Aotearoa-NZ. It is estimated that by 2038, Pacific children (aged 0–14 years) will make up almost one-fifth of all children in Aotearoa-NZ (MSD 2016; Statistics New Zealand 2016). This fast-growing population will play a pivotal role in shaping Aotearoa-NZ's economic, health and social trajectories.

Over the last 40 years, there has been an increasing presence of Māori and Pacific frameworks within Aotearoa-NZ public policy sectors such as health (HRC 2005; MOH 2018, 2020), education (MOE 2018, 2020c) and social services (MSD 2016; MPP 2018). The development of these cultural frameworks took place largely in response to concerns that the prevailing dominant approaches did not reflect the worldviews, beliefs and knowledge systems of Indigenous and Pacific people within Aotearoa-NZ public policy sectors, but rather represented Eurocentric values (see Endemann 2009; Smith 2012). The *Fonofale* model, developed by Fuimaono Karl Pulotu-Endemann (2009), is one of the most cited Pacific frameworks, and depicts Pacific peoples' understanding of health and well-being using the metaphor of a Sāmoan *fale* (house). Although the fonofale is modelled on a Sāmoan house, it includes Pacific concepts, knowledge, values and practices from many Pacific nations (Endemann 2009). The *fale*, representing one's overall well-being, has multiple interrelated elements, such as the floor, or foundation, representing *aiga* (family). The roof represents culture – the beliefs and value systems that can provide protection and shelter. The *pou* (pillars), which connect the foundation and the roof, reflect physical, spiritual, mental and other factors such as sexuality, gender and socio-economic position. These domains are encapsulated in a cocoon acknowledging that individuals and cultures experience change in relation to context, time and environment (see Figure 3.1).

A range of other models are informed by Pacific epistemologies, for example the *fa'afaletui* model (Tamasese et al. 2005). While Pacific scholars agree that no single model can provide a cultural context for all the Pacific cultures, there are commonalities across Pacific models that illustrate key shared values, such as relationships, respect and spirituality, as well as shared aspirations (Agnew et al. 2004).

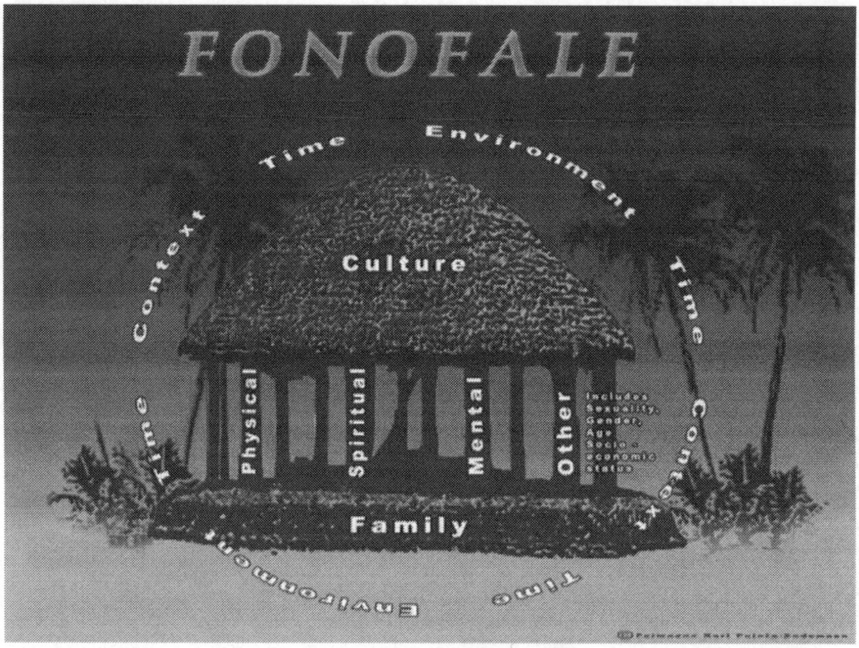


*Figure 3.1* Fonofale model (Endemann 2009, p. 3).

## Engaging Pacific concepts requires both content and process

While a number of policy and research statements describe key Pacific concepts and worldviews (see Anae et al. 2001; MOE 2018; MOH 2018) the definition of Pacific research proposed by the Health Research Council of New Zealand (HRC 2005) captures best the position that informed the writing of the nation's relationship and sexuality education policies. The Health Research Council (2005, p. 11) asserts that

> [s]ource material for Pacific health research will most likely be derived from Pacific peoples, and from within Pacific realities - past, present and future … [these] will aim to be responsive to changing Pacific contexts … [and] be underpinned by Pacific cultural values and beliefs.

In developing the relationship and sexuality education policies, Katie Fitzpatrick – the lead author of the relationships and sexuality education policy guides – was adamant that Pacific understandings would be included and written by Pacific people for Pacific communities. She formed a team with the cultural and professional expertise to ensure that Indigenous and cultural perspectives would be clearly visible and woven throughout the policy guides. These actions align with the guiding principles of engaging with Pacific peoples in Pacific Health Research

(HRC 2005). At its centre and connecting the 11 guiding principles is the cultivation and maintenance of respectful relationships (HRC 2005). Relationships are often an unexamined and unappreciated part of the policy-making process. The experience of the Pacific members in the relationships and sexuality education policy writing group contrasted markedly with reports by Pacific individuals involved in other forms of policy consultation – which is often perceived as tokenistic since, rather than at its inception Pacific input is sought only *after* a policy has been developed. Having a Pacific writing team involved from the outset, with the autonomy to review, develop and write the Pacific sections of the policies as well as input into the guide in its entirety, exemplified good practice and a deep respect for Pasifika ways.

## Pacific theories, values and contexts in policy

There are five sections in the relationship and sexuality education policy guides; Pacific understandings feature in sections one, three and five (MOE 2020a, 2020b). In the first section readers are introduced to the Aotearoa-NZ context and relationships with Pacific communities, such as the *tuakana-teina* relationship between Māori and Pacific peoples:

> Among the many concepts common to Māori and Pacific peoples is the tuakana–teina family relationship. The concept of a tuakana–teina relationship can be extended to the connection between Māori (as tāngata whenua) and Pacific people in Aotearoa New Zealand. Central features of this relationship include closeness, cooperation, mutual respect, and loyalty.
>
> (MOE 2020a, p. 14)

Contextual information such as the taboo and *tapu* (spiritual restriction) nature of discussing sexual matters, the importance of relational ties relating to Pacific communities and Pacific frameworks, including the Fonofale model, are highlighted. School communities are encouraged to explore four reflective questions that may support engagement with Pacific students and families. The third section of the policies focuses on the curriculum, where effective and empowering approaches to relationships and sexuality education for students from Pacific backgrounds are discussed. School communities are alerted to the Pacific cultural values and cultural dynamics that are likely to be present:

> Given the high regard placed on relationships within Pacific cultures and the sensitivity surrounding sexuality, schools need to recognise that discussing such issues in an open and frank manner may be very difficult for parents, ākonga [students], and teachers. Pacific values can have a huge

> bearing on how ākonga respond to the delivery of relationships and sexuality education. The cultures of Sāmoa and Tonga highlight the special relationship between a brother and sister, which has a specific code and etiquette.
>
> (MOE 2020a, p. 36)

This content sits alongside an explicit commitment in the policy guides to recognise and value non-binary approaches to gender, along with sex and sexuality diversity. The policies also acknowledge that:

> Pacific communities are diverse. Pacific people have individual identities, which include not only ethnicity, gender, and sexuality but also a host of other features. To work effectively with Pacific ākonga and their families, schools need to understand the different ways that Pacific cultures and individuals' value and express the concepts of relationship and connection.
>
> (MOE 2020a, p. 17)

Highlighting the challenges of practice (e.g. how schools can address the cultural dissonance that Pacific youth may experience when learning relationships and sexuality education alongside differently gendered peers) while also making gender diversity visible (including gender non-conformity and diversity in Pacific communities) provides an example of how the relationships and sexuality education policy is reflecting the complex policyscape from which it emerges. In this sense, these policies maintain a dynamic relationship to local understandings of gender and sexuality, framing them as complex, sometimes contradictory, but always contextual. In this respect, the acronym LGBTQI+ sits alongside MVPFAFF in the policies to denote that Western and Pacific identities are not directly translatable. While these identities are open to change, the naming of all these is explicitly included in learning statements for all young people so that *learning* about Pacific knowledges and world views is an integral part of the relationships and sexuality education curriculum.

## The intersection of policy and practice: Working with schools

To illustrate some of the possibilities and complexity of practice when delivering relationship and sexuality education with Pacific communities, it may be helpful to consider the work undertaken by the Village Collective – a Pacific non-governmental organisation comprising Pacific sexual health promoters who aim to equip young people, families and communities with the knowledge and resources to achieve good sexual health. Part of the collective's work lies in supporting schools to deliver culturally responsive education to Pacific youth. The *Navig8 Program* case vignette, discussed, demonstrates how the collective engages with gender and sexuality issues in school settings. This account of the Collective's experience with school communities reflects how relationships and sexuality education policies intersect with school-based programmes in ways that can promote and value Pacific epistemologies. This is particularly important as the structural and philosophical frameworks underpinning many Aotearoa-NZ schools are driven by Western models of education. When working with Pacific communities, it is important to understand some of the key concepts which underpin Pacific practices. *Vā* and *talanoa* are foundational principles.

Vā or *va* is a term common to Tonga (vā) and Samoa (va) and describes relational connections between people or people and places like the land, sky and ocean. *Tauhi vā* is a Tongan term that describes the act and principles when taking care of others and oneself, and is viewed as a reciprocal exchange. In delivering relationships and sexuality education school-based programmes, the Village Collective appreciate several layers of vā. These include the vā between the external provider and the school, the vā (and responsibilities) of the school with their students and families, the vā between the provider and the students and their families, and the vā between students themselves. When delivering sexuality education sessions, demonstrating gender inclusivity without compromising notions of vā can be complex.

As Pacific educators and health promoters, talanoa is one of the many ways Pacific peoples connect. Rooted in oral traditions, talanoa is a process recognised in many Pacific nations. As Pacific contributors, we would describe talanoa as an unconscious learned practice — a natural way of relating, of sharing and connecting. Talanoa involves a deep, interpersonal exchange of emotional and cultural sharing between all the storytellers and the listeners (Vaioleti 2006).

## *Engaging the vā/va and gender inclusion*

### *Initial Talanoa sessions*

In their initial meeting with school management and nominated staff, the Village Collective explores the school's aims and aspirations for relationships and sexuality education delivery, noting the strengths and challenges with existing approaches. Connections with families and local communities are also examined, particularly as the New Zealand Education and Training Act 2020 requires schools to consult with their community (MoE 2020a). The Village Collective then discusses *Navig8*, their comprehensive drama-based relationship education programme for primary and intermediate students. As part of building engagement with Pacific parents and their families, the collective encourages school management to hold a talanoa session in which the team discuss the programme in Pacific languages, using Pacific metaphors. This talanoa with school management and families lays the foundations on which future relationships can be built.

The parent and family talanoa session is often co-facilitated with school staff. Interactive approaches are a popular method for engaging Pacific parents and their children. Attendees have the choice of participating in small group discussions, the composition of which is determined by those in attendance. For example, some may prefer joining an ethnic-specific group (i.e. Samoan or Tongan), a gender group (assigned male at birth/assigned female at birth) or a family role group (mother/father/grandparents/children). The Village Collective team is acutely aware that the option of biological sex groups may create an unsafe environment for gender non-conforming and diverse participants. So, from the outset, the team takes care to ensure that the group processes reflect the universal value of *fa'aloalo* (respect) and the acceptance of vā (the relationships between participants).

One example of an interactive approach that has proved especially popular with Pacific parents is the 'pubertal changes matching activity.' In this activity, participants are provided with information cards that describe the mental, emotional and physical changes to expect during puberty, such as 'mood swings' or 'periods begin.' They then need to match if these are experienced by males, females or both. The pubertal changes matching activity aims to teach participants about the physical bodies they are born into, that for some people their physical body does not match their identity and that some changes are sex-specific while others are not.

For the parents of some gender non-conforming and diverse children, the idea of a sex-segregated puberty session may amplify fears that their children may experience further alienation and bullying. Some parents worry that the puberty sessions may assert messages such as 'turn back to God' or 'just be a boy.' Young fakaleitī have confidently shared: 'I know it's not gonna be about people telling me to be a boy, but about how to look after the body I have now …' and as a result, are happy to be part of a 'male' group.

### *Navig8 programme*

The Village Collective's *Navig8* programme for primary and intermediate students consists of six, one-hour workshops that draw on a holistic approach of engaging and connecting. Although there have been some advances in the field of sexuality education, the terms 'sex' or 'sexuality' continue to raise much distress and confusion, particularly amongst Pacific parents. In *Navig8* work, the term 'relationships' is used to allow opportunities to explore the myriad of issues in relation to sexuality. The first two workshops focus on 'respect' and 'friendships,' and aim to build rapport with students and identify existing knowledge and attitudes towards relationships (the vā). Sessions three and four are sexuality education workshops that explore 'pubertal changes' and the 'human reproductive system.' The final two workshops, 'support' and 'keeping safe online,' are aimed at equipping students with help-seeking skills and knowledge.

The success of these workshops is largely determined by the safe, accepting and open space created by the facilitators. Prior to launching in and discussing issues such as diverse gender and sexual identities, the team ensures students gain a sense of belonging in the group, that students recognise the similarities and differences amongst themselves, and that the students recognise that difference, in its many forms, is okay. Furthermore, in their talanoa with students and their families, the Collective aims to ensure that the *mana* (dignity) of those involved, such as students, are recognised and enhanced.

Students remain in their usual class group for four of the six workshops: respect, friendships, support, and keeping safe online. For the puberty workshops, students participate in either an assigned male at birth group, or an assigned female at birth group. The collective team uses the term 'gender-split' to describe the groups as there is great variation in Pacific parents' understanding of terms such as 'gender diverse' and 'rainbow.' Terms such as assigned male or female at birth are not commonly understood in school and Pacific communities. On most occasions, two male Village Collective staff will facilitate the assigned male at birth group and two female staff will facilitate the assigned female at birth group. Across the Pacific, as elsewhere, many schools continue to separate students into 'boy' and 'girl' groups. The practice of directing young people into such groups is accepted in many Pacific communities, particularly when there may be discussion of sexual content or exposure to sexual imagery. This practice stems from the principle of respecting the vā – the space between two individuals, and in the case of relationship and sexuality education, is particularly relevant when students may be in the same class as a family member of the opposite binary gender.

A mixed gender group option is also offered to all students and the sessions are facilitated by Collective staff who identify as gender non-binary and/or gender and or sexuality diverse. In order to support gender non-conforming and diverse students, the collective team has identified school locations where gender non-conforming and diverse students feel most safe and who, at home and school, are the key support people are for these students. These supporters are invited to the initial talanoa session alongside the students' parents. Overall feedback from students and staff is highly complimentary of the Village Collective facilitators and the *Navig8* programme. Students report that they are able to identify with the Village Collective team, and that the team are able to connect, communicate and create an open and safe environment for talanoa.

As this account demonstrates, delivering relationship and sexuality education with Pacific communities requires skills in engagement, cultural understandings of sexuality, as well as an understanding of the contemporary issues facing Pacific young people. These examples illustrate the value of early and ongoing conversations between schools and the importance of building good relationships with Pacific parents before relationships and sexuality education classes. These conversations and approaches are just a small beginning towards engaging Pacific worldviews into Western education.

## Conclusion: Policy and practice for Pacific relationships and sexuality education

Improving the sexual health, well-being and learning of Pacific communities is a complex endeavour requiring input and support from multiple partners and commitment at various levels (individuals, families and communities, local and central government). Official government policy documents, such as the Aotearoa-NZ relationship and sexuality policy guides, provide an opportunity to inform future practice. The writing team responsible for developing current relationships and sexuality education policies (MOE 2020a, 2020b) was committed to making Pacific concepts visible, especially those of greatest relevance to communities in Aotearoa-NZ.

The policies are now official Government documents and the Pacific concepts they contain have been given official government recognition and status. This is significant in a country which continues to deal with an ongoing inheritance of colonisation. As demonstrated here, engaging in policy (and practice) can be complex because it requires seemingly static curriculum policy documents to engage with some of the contradictions and cultural nuances of the policyscape from which they emerge. Further research that captures how Pacific concepts and values can inform relationships and sexuality education policy and practice, such as vā/va and talanoa, are necessary. Only in this way can relationships and sexuality education policy respond to global, local and cultural contexts whilst re-imagining future possibilities. Central government agencies, such as the Ministry of Education, have a key role to play in this respect. Sustained commitment to, and prioritisation of, Indigenous and Pacific knowledge in government policy is a necessary step to realising good sexual and reproductive health and well-being for all members of society. As the Honourable Aupito Tofae Su'a William Sio, Minister for Pacific Peoples recently stated, 'What is good for Pacific peoples is good for Aotearoa New Zealand' (MPP 2018, p. 4).

## Notes

1 The authors of this chapter were part of the writing team for the new relationships and sexuality education guides. Katie, the lead writer from the University of Auckland, engaged Analosa (University of Auckland) and Riki from the Village Collective to collaborate in reviewing the existing guide and updating content for Pacific communities.

2 State-integrated are schools with a 'special character.' They may be run by a particular religious faith, e.g. Catholic, or use specialist education methods, such as Steiner and Montessori schools.

## References

Allen, L. and Rasmussen, M.L., 2016. *The Palgrave handbook of sexuality education*. London: Palgrave Macmillan.

Agnew, F., et al., 2004. *Pacific models of mental health service delivery in New Zealand: ("PMMHSD") project*. Auckland: Health Research Council of New Zealand.

Anae, M., et al., 2001. *Pasifika education research guidelines*. Wellington: Ministry of Education.

Ball, S.J., Maguire, M., and Braun, A., 2012. *How schools do policy: Policy enactments in secondary schools*. Abingdon: Routledge.

Clark, T.C., et al., 2014. The health and well-being of transgender high school students: Results from the New Zealand Adolescent Health Survey (Youth'12). *Journal of Adolescent Health*, 55 (1), 93–99. doi:10.1016/j.jadohealth.2013.11.008

Endemann, F.K., 2009. *Fonofale model of health*. Available from: https://www.mpp.govt.nz/assets/Resources/Fonofale-presentation-to-Pacific-Wellbeing-Talanoa-May-2021.pdf [Accessed 14 October 2021].

Farran, S., 2010. Pacific perspectives: Fa'afafine and Fakaleiti in Samoa and Tonga: People between worlds. *Liverpool Law Review*, 31 (1), 13–28.

Fenaughty, J. et al., 2021. *Transgender and diverse gender students: A Youth 19 brief*. Youth19, 11 April. Available from: https://www.youth19.ac.nz/publications [Accessed 1 September 2021].

HRC, 2005. *Guidelines on Pacific health research*. Auckland: Health Research Council of New Zealand.

MOE, 2018. *Tapasa cultural competencies framework for teachers of Pacific learners*. Wellington: Ministry of Education. Available from: https://pasifika.tki.org.nz/Tapasa [Accessed 1 September 2021].

MOE, 2020a. *Relationships and sexuality education. A guide for teachers, leaders, and boards of trustees. Years 1-8*. Wellington: Ministry of Education. Available from: https://health.tki.org.nz/Teaching-in-HPE/Policy-Guidelines/Relationships-and-Sexuality-Education [Accessed 1 September 2021].

MOE, 2020b. *Relationships and sexuality education. A guide for teachers, leaders, and boards of trustees. Years 9-13*. Wellington: Ministry of Education. Available: https://health.tki.org.nz/Teaching-in-HPE/Policy-Guidelines/Relationships-and-Sexuality-Education [Accessed 1 September 2021].

MOE, 2020c. *Action plan for Pacific education*. Wellington: Ministry of Education. Available from: https://conversation.education.govt.nz/conversations/action-plan-for-pacific-education/ [Accessed 1 September 2021].

MOH, 2018.*'Ala Mo'ui progress report: Pacific health care utilisation*. Wellington: Ministry of Health.

MOH, 2020. *Ola Manuia: Pacific health and wellbeing action plan. 2020-2025*. Wellington: Ministry of Health, 13 June. Available from: https://www.health.govt.nz/publication/ola-manuia-pacific-health-and-wellbeing-action-plan-2020-2025 [Accessed 1 September 2021].

MPP, 2018. *Pacific Aotearoa. Lalanga Fou*. Wellington: Ministry for Pacific Peoples. https://www.mpp.govt.nz/assets/Reports/Pacific-Aotearoa-Lalanga-Fou-Report.pdf [Accessed 14 October 2021].

MSD, 2016. *The profile of Pacific peoples in New Zealand. September 2016. Pasefika Proud Resource*. Wellington: Ministry of Social Development. Available from: https://www.pasefikaproud.co.nz/assets/Resources-for-download/PasefikaProudResource-Pacific-peoples-paper.pdf [Accessed 1 September 2021].

Mundy, K., et al., 2016. *The handbook of global education policy*. Chichester, UK: John Wiley & Sons.

Pulotu-Endemann F.K. and Peteru, M.C., 2001. Beyond the paradise myth: Sexuality and identity. In: C. Macpherson, P. Spoonley and M. Anae (eds), *Tangata O Te Moana Nui. The evolving identities of Pacific peoples in Aotearoa/New Zealand*. Palmerston North: Dunmore Press, 122–136.

Smith, L., 1999. *Decolonizing methodologies: Research and indigenous peoples*. Dunedin: University of Otago Press.

Smith, L., 2012. *Decolonizing methodologies: Research and indigenous peoples*. 2nd ed. London, New York: Zed Books.

Statistics New Zealand, 2016. *National ethnic population projections: 2013(base)–2038*. Wellington: Statistics New Zealand. Available from: http://www.stats.govt.nz [Accessed 1 September 2021].

Statistics New Zealand, 2019. *New Zealand's population reflects growing diversity*. Wellington: Statistics New Zealand, 23 September. Available from: https://www.stats.govt.nz/news/new-zealands-population-reflects-growing-diversity [Accessed 1 September 2021].

Tamasese, K., et al., 2005. Ole Taeao Afua, the new morning: A qualitative investigation into Samoan perspectives on mental health and culturally appropriate services. *Australian and New Zealand Journal of Psychiatry*, 39 (4), 300–309.

Vaioleti, T.M., 2006. Talanoa research methodology: A developing position on Pacific research. *Waikato Journal of Education*, 12, 21–34.

Veukiso-Ulugia, A., 2012. *Best practice framework for the delivery of sexual health promotion services to Pacific communities in New Zealand*. Available from: https://tewhariki.org.nz/assets/best-practice-sexual-health-framework-for-pacific-people-final-170kb.pdf [Accessed 1 September 2021].

# 4 Inangaro | Desire: The 'writing in' of māpū | young Cook Islanders' sexual and relationship desires into resources for sexuality and relationships education

*Debi Futter-Puati*

## Introduction

Often grounded in colonialist Western ideas, education provision for māpū | young people in the Pacific is influenced by international trends and is rarely contextualised to the local setting. This is particularly the situation for sex, sexuality and relationships education. Drawing on the socio-cultural knowledge of young people in the Kuki Airani | Cook Islands, this chapter seeks discuss the issues this raises for sex, sexuality and relationships education by exploring māpū | young people's experiences about these matters. This māpū | youth-grounded knowledge was used for the development of a culturally relevant Kuki Airani educational resource for both school and community settings.

## The Kuki Airani: Context

The Kuki Airani[1] | Cook Islands is an independent nation situated in the South Pacific Ocean, northeast of Aotearoa | New Zealand (Aotearoa-NZ), between Tahiti and Fiji. The country is a 'large ocean state' (Reeves 2012) comprising 15 islands spread across 2.2 million square kilometres of ocean. Approximately 15,000 people populate the country (Cook Islands Ministry of Finance and Economic Management 2016), with 74% of the population residing in Rarotonga, the main island. Most residents are Kuki Airani Māori (86%), with a significant diaspora of Kuki Airani living in Aotearoa-NZ and in Australia.

Historically, Ariki | paramount chiefs were the leaders of the Kuki Airani. In pre-Christian times, the spiritual and physical dimensions of life were inseparable, involving many rituals, rites, ceremonies, and prayers associated with everyday experiences (Buck 1939; Crocombe and Holmes 2014). Arriving in 1821, the London Missionary Society missionaries from French Polynesia (formerly Tahiti and the Society Islands) introduced Christianity and within a short time Christianity had a strong influence, which remains in the present day.[2] Given the very high proportion of the population who are members of a Christian-based religion, adherence to Christianity has become a central tenet of everyday life. In 1888, the Kuki Airani was colonised by Britain and declared

DOI: 10.4324/9781003142072-5

a protectorate of the British Crown, and in 1901 the country was annexed to Aotearoa-NZ. The postcolonial period[3] for the Kuki Airani began in 1965 when the country became self-governing but in free association with Aotearoa-NZ.[4] The impact of colonisation did not end however, when the colonising body withdrew (Childs and Williams 2013). As the concept of neo-colonialism articulates, 'Western powers were still intent on exercising and maintaining maximum indirect control over erstwhile colonies via political, cultural and above all, economic channels' (Childs and Williams 2013, p. 5). In the name of 'development,' agencies such as the Secretariat of the Pacific Community and United Nations organisations including UNFPA, UNESCO and the World Health Organization, and others involved with sex/sexuality/relationships education in the Pacific, can exert neo-colonialistic influence (Vai'imene 2003).

## Tuatua 'Akamat'anga | Introducing the research project

Some academics working in Indigenous settings fall short in their appreciation and understanding of the standards of relational accountability expected of them as researchers by the communities in which they undertake research (Smith 2012; Kelly-Hanku et al. 2021). Not engaging Indigenous people fully within the research process is increasingly brought into question, including in the Pacific. Kelly-Hanku et al. (2021) contend that in Papua New Guinea Indigenous people have often not been consulted about research that is done on and about them: they have historically been researched on, and rarely included in the analysis. In more recent years, with efforts in research capacity building and decolonial approaches to research, including global health, this has shifted with a transition from what they call 'the researched to the researchers' (Kelly-Hanku et al. 2021). Writing against the dominant deficit discourse of academic research in Indigenous societies, the Maori anthropologist Linda Tuhiwai Smith (2012) also notes the need for research that focuses on the agency and potential of Indigenous communities. She argues that it is only by drawing on the cultural strengths and understandings that communities have of themselves that communities can lead their own transformation.

As a long-term resident of Kuki Airani who is deeply connected with families and communities through marriage, family and enduring relationships, I have sought to honour an Indigenous worldviews approach in the work discussed here. I used a Kuki Airani research framework called the Tivaevae framework, to explore sex, sexuality and relationships education with māpū | youth in the Kuki Airani (for more on the Tivaevae framework see Futter-Puati and Maua-Hodges 2019). Developed by Teremoana Maua-Hodges, the Tivaevae framework borrows from the traditions and processes of creating a traditional Tivaevae | handmade quilt (see Figure 4.1), and seeks to represent Kuki Airani epistemological and ontological worldviews (Futter-Puati and Maua-Hodges 2019).

The use of the Tivaevae framework ensured the research method I chose empowered māpū by using their own knowledge and experience(s) of sex, relationship and sexuality education, and to identify their own needs. Findings

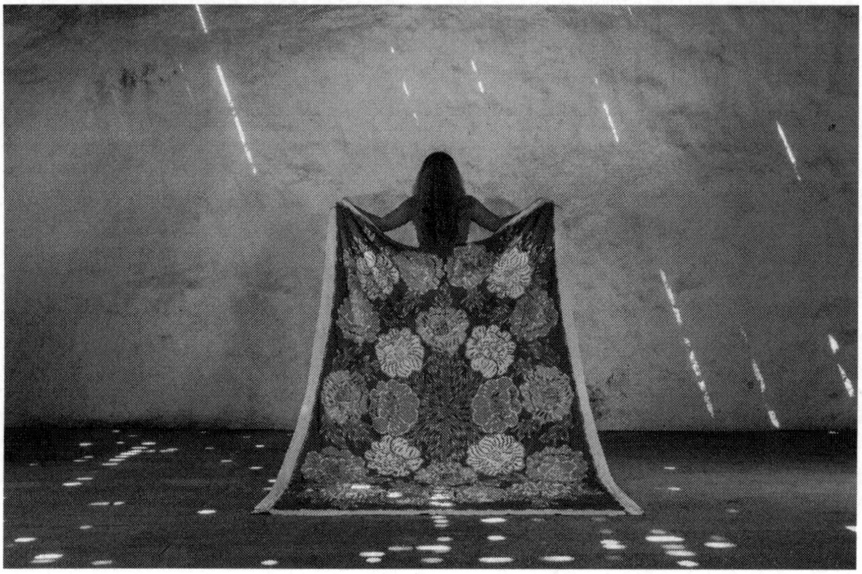

*Figure 4.1* Example of Tivaevae. Created and sewed by unknown. Photo by Melanie Cooper.

from the research showed clearly that the design of sex, sexuality and relationships education needs to be culturally relevant, but at the same time, it should take a strengths-based and sex-positive approach; the latter frequently being perceived by older people as provocative and non-Kuki Airani.

Kuki Airani māpū wanted their education to focus on their abilities, strengths and needs, rather than on how they are often 'framed' by adults: as irresponsible and in need of protection. Such imaginings of māpū fail to understand how māpū embrace and straddle multi-cultures at the same time. The educational resource endeavoured to make available the knowledge and skills māpū identified; they needed to navigate the environment(s) they find themselves in, rather than what has traditionally been offered — in the form of a situation in which adults decide what they need or 'should' do. In this way, and by taking a Tivaevae approach, the resource supports māpū while pushing boundaries, and challenging wider Kuki Airani adult and traditional understandings of sex education and the lives of māpū.

## Sexuality approaches in the Pacific

Similar to many Western countries, the Pacific has historically adopted a medicalised public health approach to sexual and reproductive health and education. This imported approach emphasises reducing 'risk' by seeking to address individual behaviour. Programmes are often designed and implemented from within a biomedical perspective so lack of attention to environmental and structural conditions is not unsurprising. Most usually, the focus is on HIV and sexually transmitted infection (STI) prevention and the prevention of teenage pregnancy from within a heterocentric framework. For example, the Family Life Education programme in Fiji was designed for school children with the aim of reducing pregnancies among young people as well as HIV and STIs, but did so within a conservative, medicalised, risk reduction and abstinence-based model (Naz 2014; Varani-Norton 2014).

Another focus of sexuality education has been to ensure young people remain productive and contributing members of society while protecting the limited resources of Pacific nations from overpopulation (Secretariat of the Pacific Community 2010). For instance, the Aotearoa-NZ Parliamentarians' Group on Population and Development recommended the following:

> … if the youth of the Pacific don't get access to good sexual reproductive health services and education, that population's going to explode in the next generation or two and the environment in their own country wouldn't be able to sustain greater population. It's actually urgent; it's more than urgent.
>
> (Radio New Zealand 2012)

The above comment confirms that anxiety derives not only from biomedical and public health priorities, but also from concerns about sustainability. As a result, māpū in Kuki Airani and the Pacific more generally have become the target of many health-related interventions, often instigated and/or funded by outside development organisations. Until recently, the focus has mainly been on HIV and STI prevention, with resources being designed by several organisations for use throughout the Pacific (Secretariat of the Pacific Community 2010). Evidence has shown this kind of generic approach to programming is ineffective, as catering to context is vital to success (see, for example, Thammaraksa et al. 2014; Blake and Aggleton 2016).

## Akaruru | Data generation

The purpose of the research project described in this chapter was to develop a culturally appropriate educational resource for use in Kuki Airani that was driven by the needs of māpū (see Futter-Puati 2017b). Using the traditions and processes employed to create a traditional tivaevae, the research exegesis (Futter-Puati 2017a) and project (Futter-Puati 2017b) were written in such a way to create a metaphorical tivaevae in honour of, and symbolising, māpū views of their sexuality landscape. In order to be able to gain a deep understanding of the complexity and contradictions of māpū lives, both qualitative and quantitative research methods were utilised.

Designed in consultation with māpū and the Ministry of Health, a self-administered anonymous questionnaire was used to examine perspectives on sex and sexuality and the relationships māpū have, or would like to have. The use of a self-administered electronic questionnaire offered an opportunity to ask questions not previously asked of māpū in the Kuki Airani, questions that are frequently deemed culturally inappropriate or which participants might struggle to answer openly if asked by a researcher. A total of 674 māpū, aged between 15 and 24 years, completed the survey, accounting for more than 20% of the māpū population across all of the populated islands at that time. Six focus group discussions were also held to provide māpū the opportunity to discuss issues in greater depth and to elicit peer and community perspectives on sexuality. One of these groups was exclusively akava'ine | boys and men who identify and seek to live as girls or women.

Analysis of the questionnaire and focus group data was undertaken using the lenses provided by feminist poststructural and postcolonial theory to explore culture, identity, power, agency, gender, performativity and heteronormativity (Davies 2000; Butler 2004; Jackson and Mazzei 2012; Smith 2012). Analysing and examining the data through these approaches to identify the way māpū discursively constituted sexuality in the Kuki Airani facilitated a critical understanding of these aspects of Kuki Airani life.

## Akatomo'anga | Findings

Apart from the boys in one outer island focus group, all other māpū documented the importance of, and need to, include content that addresses sexuality and gender diversity and transgender. In fact, they insisted on it. The insistence from māpū that these issues be included in future programmes was significant in shaping the resource that was produced as an outcome of the research. Each of the focus group discussions recounted stories of either experiencing or witnessing sexual and verbal violence and/or discrimination against akava'ine, māpū at school and in the community and many described how they felt uncomfortable and helpless to know how to respond.

| | |
|---|---|
| *Sarah:* | I would be called 'cocksucker' all day at school but as soon as the sun sets, they want their cocks sucked ... so what did I do? I did it. I just do it to them as next time I have something to throw back at them[5] |
| *Serena:* | We were talking about DNA and genes and things, you know XY and XX ... the high school teacher told this other person in the class: 'You are an XXY ... can you stand up and say what being akava'ine is like'? |
| *Interviewer:* | So, he totally humiliated you in front of the class? |
| *Serena:* | Yes |

Significantly, 23% of the participants in the questionnaire were unwilling or chose not to identify their sexuality or gender. This may be linked to concern about possible victimisation or discrimination that has been the experience of other people of diverse sexualities and or gender identities including in Kuki Airani (Besnier and Alexeyeff 2014). The internalised impact of the discriminatory practices against people in Kuki Airani whose sexuality and gender challenges hegemonic heteronormativity can be seen in the high number of calls received by the local suicide prevention helpline regarding sexual orientation and gender identity (Cook Islands Ministry of Internal Affairs: Youth Suicide Prevention Steering Committee 2015).

The level of support offered by participants across all but one of the focus groups for the inclusion of sexuality and gender diversity and gender nonconformity provides insights into the strongly held values many of today's māpū, and their concern for social justice and human rights. One young woman, Teata, explained her appreciation of social justice and awareness of the potential impact of not addressing sexual diversity in sexuality education for those who may be lesbian, gay, bisexual or transgender.

> ... you know, it doesn't mean to say that you are homosexual if you are learning about homosexuality. But if you are gay, then it's good to know that other people might feel like that too, and that it's not just you ... that you are not on your own.

Despite the popular perception that the Pacific, and particularly Polynesia, is a safe and accepting space for akava'ine, māpū were very aware of the limited acceptance of akava'ine, and disturbed by witnessing how akava'ine are treated, suggesting that akava'ine are only accepted superficially. Within a focus group of akava'ine everyone nodded in agreement when Vaine commented, 'You are accepted as a woman to clean the house, babysit, cook ... but you are not allowed a male partner.' The influence of conservative Christianity was blamed by participants for this limited acceptance, with māpū seeing through the 'so called' acceptance of the transgender community in the Kuki Airani.

Almost all of the participants in the survey (93%) had experienced vaginal or anal sex on at least one occasion, and of these, 40% percent had had their sexual debut before 14 years of age. Although the median age of first sex for girls/young women was 15, the median age of sexual debut for boys/young men was 14. In focus group discussions, māpū confirmed that early sexual debut was common. Moreover, while almost all participants responded that they had knowledge of how to use a condom conversely, only 42% reported doing so at their first sexual experience. These data indicate a gap between 'knowing' and 'doing' which is common in other contexts (Cook Islands Ministry of Health and Secretariat of the Pacific Community 2007; Varani-Norton 2014; Iyler and Aggleton 2015), and could be linked to condom accessibility in a conservative community.

Māpū discussed the challenges they experienced from peers if they were not sexually active early in their teenage years. Beyond peer pressure, there was coercion to deal with as illustrated in the text that follows from a mixed gender focus group of 15–20-year-olds in Rarotonga, and who were part of a youth peer support group at a non-governmental organisation.

*Interviewer:* So, explain to me why young people get into relationships?
*Tiare:* 'cause you are forced to
*Interviewer:* Do you mean you are forced to do something sexual, or forced how?
*Tiare:* I don't want to answer that question.
*Interviewer:* Okay. So, [to the rest of the group] sometimes you are forced to go out with someone, or have sex with someone?
*Marama:* Yeah - sometimes you're forced to go out with someone
*Telaina:* Yeah 'cause everyone else is
*Interviewer:* So does that mean that you 'should' be as well?
*Marama:* Yeah
*Interviewer:* So, you do it to keep up with your friends even though you might not want to?
*Consensus:* Yeah

While there was pressure from peers to be sexually active, the reverse was true from parents and caregivers. Māpū shared on many occasions how fearful they were at their parents finding out they were sexually active. They typically only told their parents they were sexually active when something went wrong (e.g. pregnancy), and they needed their help. After learning their child was sexually active, some māpū were rejected by their families, were forced to marry and live with their sexual partner, were sent away from their home to live with family overseas or, in the worst case, subjected to physical violence.

Ripeka's experience was not untypical: 'I wasn't allowed to go out with boys and it wasn't until I got pregnant that they found out I was … [sexually active]. [That] is when the family stepped in … .' At the time she got pregnant, Repeka's family afforded her little to no autonomy. She had to sneak out to be with her boyfriend. Once her pregnancy became known she was made to stay at home. But in practice her situation was very different to that of her boyfriend. Highlighting the inequalities in parental responsibility between herself and her boyfriend she continued:

> … but he didn't feel like he should listen. They wanted us both at home, but soon after that he was going out. We had this newborn family and he was going out and my family had to step in … but he didn't listen to my parents and do something … he knows when he goes out, knowing he does all that he wants [have sex with others], and he knows at the back of his mind: whatever I do tonight I will still have my baby and my girlfriend.

## Fresh ways to (re)consider sexuality and relationships education in the Pacific

Overall, findings from this study reveal the need to develop an educational resource informed by māpū realities and using a sex-positive approach. Almost all participants identified themselves as sexual subjects/sexually active in the ways they responded to the questionnaire as well as in the focus group discussions. That most māpū were sexually active before the age of 14 reinforced this view, as did their descriptions of sex outside of committed relationships and concurrent sexual relationships. This new knowledge provided context to inform the development of teaching and learning materials that are contextually relevant and engage with sexuality and gender diversity among other concerns. It also signposted that if sexual and relationships education were to be meaningful, māpū require multiple opportunities to consider, learn and practise skills of critical thinking, decision-making, problem solving, negotiation and communication in sexual situations (Ollis 2015).

Acknowledging in an education resource that high school student māpū are sexually active was potentially contentious with most of the mainly conservative Kuki Airani adult community, as it challenged heteronormative, cultural, and patriarchal discourses of māpū sexual lives (Smith and Gunn 2015). To deal with this I piloted a series of 20 lessons based on key findings from the data. These were trialled with two groups. One of adult educators from school and community settings, from across multiple islands and the other, a group of māpū, to gauge their responses. The adult educators reported feeling challenged in the weeklong experience, particularly regarding their knowledge and understanding as well as values on matters of sexual and gender diversity and multiple relationships. The week gave these adults, educated members of the community, the chance to review the research and understand the need(s) of māpū which underpinned the lessons. By the end of the week the evaluations indicated strong support of the resource with minor adaptions mainly to ensure the activities aligned with Kuki Airani cultural context. Informed by what I learned from this process, I further developed an engaging, sex-positive resource for use by educators that reflect the sexual lives of māpū. This resource would support the sexuality education which is mandated for all schools in the Cook Islands Oraanga e te Tupuanga Meitaki | Health and Physical Wellbeing curriculum (2006). This curriculum document was developed through a nationwide consultation process in which each island community identified sexuality as an important context to be taught to māpū.

Once the resource was published all community and school sexuality educators received a copy and underwent a weeklong training in the use of the resource. This professional development opportunity also included four sexuality educator mentors (two from community non-government settings and two from school settings) to co-facilitate the training and be available for schools and non-governmental organisations to support their implementation of the resource in their own settings. Findings from earlier discussion with māpū themselves signalled the need to incorporate activities into sexuality and relationships education that triggered discussion about whether or not 'taking risks' might be 'worth it' (Gilbert 2014), which for many in Kuki Airani educators was another contentious approach as it raised the ideas of the previously missing discourse of desire and pleasure within sexuality education (Fine 1988).

## About the sexuality and relationships educational resource

The aim of the resource was for māpū who were taught the lessons to develop the skills and knowledge to be able to enjoy equitable, responsible, fulfilling and healthy sexual lives. The lessons envisioned supporting māpū to develop critical thinking skills in relation to sexuality and relationships that would enable them to understand six imperative themes. These were: that they are actively involved in the construction of their sexuality and gender identity; that there is a wide range of difference and diversity within all groups related to sex, gender and relationships; to understand how discriminatory practices can damage the well-being of themselves and others; how societal influences and power structures operate in the construction of sexuality and gender; how to challenge restrictions placed on them by others' constructions of gender and/or sexuality; and ultimately the resource hoped to enable skills to become a sexually healthy adult.[6]

Each lesson begins with the rationale for the lesson via a link to the findings of the research undertaken with māpū. Linking findings of the research to each individual lesson created identifications of the need for each lesson for the educators. This link became especially important for lessons that had not been recognised as needed previously. One example is described below.

When discussing the difficulties they experienced in relationships, every focus group described the normalcy of both adult and māpū multiple and concurrent relationships. Most often a discussion around fidelity ensued and discussion of the emotional, and sometimes physical, altercations that arose from finding out their partner was 'cheating.' Given the frequency of concurrent relationships in the Kuki Airani, much consideration was given to how concurrent relationships could be undertaken in a way that was safe and in which reduced the level of emotional and physical violence apparent in the lives of participants when partners were found to be cheating. This led to the inclusion of a lesson about polyamorous (multi-partner) relationships within the programme (see Futter-Puati 2017b, pp. 122–123). The lesson explores the idea that some people may want to have more than one relationship at the same time and that polyamorous people openly engage in romantic/sexual relationships with multiple people concurrently, with the emphasis on long-term intimate relationships with a focus on honesty (Sheff 2005).[7] The use of such a scenario aims to stimulate critical thinking about alternatives to the way in which concurrent relationships are currently experienced. Students debate and consider why concurrent relationships occur, as well as who is advantaged or disadvantaged, when such relationships are entered into without open communication. Such a learning opportunity provides māpū with the chance to analyse hegemonic heterosexual monogamous marriage expectations alongside other normalised practices of multiple concurrent albeit, 'secretive' relationships. Completing such activities could support māpū to consider what type(s) of relationships they may, or may not, wish to participate in, and how to communicate this sensitively to others.

The international literature on comprehensive and on-going sexuality and relationships education repeatedly shows that in addition to knowledge, it is important – even more so – to develop the skills and strategies of young people to be emotionally, mentally, and physically safe within their relationships (Iyler and Aggleton 2015). In order for this to happen, educators must understand and appreciate the contexts in which the māpū they teach live and negotiate issues of sex, relationships and sexuality. It is imperative therefore to have a good understanding of the lived experiences and cultural contexts māpū find themselves in. Drawing on the findings in this research, future education about sex, sexuality and relationships in the Pacific needs to provide multiple opportunities to safely explore complex, competing and emerging beliefs, values, practices and moral frameworks. Providing opportunities to help māpū explore alternative viewpoints to hegemonic discourse is important, particularly where church doctrine, adult authority, and particular narratives of what is culturally appropriate dominate.

One possibility explored in the educational resource in the Kuki Airani was to create a culturally relevant critical reflection tool which can be used after each lesson (see Futter-Puati, 2017b, p. 132). The reflection tool has māpū reflect on what they have considered in each lesson related to the range of influences they are surrounded by. It then asks them to decide where they stand *at that point in time* on the given topic of the lesson. There are no right or wrong answers. In this way they are processing and reflecting on their values and beliefs that can support and guide them in their choices and practices.

This research project set out to understand the sexuality and relationships context of māpū in the Kuki Airani. My hopes for this research were that the findings would be taken seriously and help to reimagine sexuality and relationships education and how it could be delivered in the Pacific. By basing the resource on the lived realities, and self-identified needs, of māpū (a proviso that young Cook Islanders are not naïve and without agency as they are sometimes (mis)understood to be) the project identified a solution to designing a needs-led resource that is contextually appropriate. As it is being implemented in community settings, as well as schools, sexuality and relationships education has the potential to impact positively on the lives of māpū. Comments have been shared with me by educators who are implementing the lessons with māpū in the Kuki Airani. These educators have expressed the significant learning they themselves have experienced with implementing the teaching and learning from this resource as well as the engagement of the māpū they work with. Without an evaluation it is difficult to say if behaviours have changed but if even a few seeds of change have been sown through the educational resource, then one does have to hope.

## Notes

1 Kuki Airani Maori is the first language of the Cook Islands. Cook Islands words will not be italicised, so as not to 'other' Kuki Airani Maori language in relation to English. When writing both Kuki Airani Maori and English words a ' | ' will be used rather than a traditional '/' so as not to favour one language over another. Thereafter the first time a Kuki Airani Maori word is used there will be an English translation; subsequently Maori will be used.

2 There are now many denominations in the country such as the Cook Islands Christian Church, formerly the LMS and the predominant denomination (49% of the population), Catholic (next most popular), Seventh Day Adventist, Mormon, Latter Day Saints, Baha'i and other apostolic religions (Cook Islands Ministry of Finance and Economic Management 2012).
3 The period coming after the end of colonialism (Childs and Williams 2013).
4 Being 'in free association with Aotearoa-NZ' describes the unique arrangement between these two countries that allows Cook Islanders to maintain Aotearoa-NZ citizenship while at the same time being free to make their own laws and control their own constitution (Ministry of Foreign Affairs and Trade 2021).
5 Others in the group agreed that they would take the same action in order to have something to use back against the perpetrators of the bullying.
6 Defined as an adult who can: Appreciate one's own body; Seek further information about reproduction as needed; Affirm that human development includes sexual development, which may or may not include reproduction or sexual experience; Interact with all genders in respectful and appropriate ways; Affirm one's own sexual orientation and respect the sexual orientations of others; Affirm one's own gender identities and respect the gender identities of others; Express love and intimacy in appropriate ways; Develop and maintain meaningful relationships; Avoid exploitative or manipulative relationships; Make informed choices about family options and relationships; Exhibit skills that enhance personal relationships; Identify and live according to one's own values; Take responsibility for one's own behaviour; Practice effective decision-making; Develop critical-thinking skills; Communicate effectively with family, peers, and sexual partners; Enjoy and express one's sexuality throughout life; Express one's sexuality in ways that are compatible with one's values; Enjoy sexual feelings without necessarily acting on them; Discriminate between life-enhancing sexual behaviours and those that are harmful to self and/or others; Express one's sexuality while respecting the rights of others; Seek new information to enhance one's sexuality; Engage in sexual relationships that are consensual, non-exploitative, honest, pleasurable and protected; Practice health-promoting behaviours, such as regular sexual health check-ups, breast and testicular self-exam and early identification of potential problems; Use contraception effectively to avoid unintended pregnancy; Avoid contracting or transmitting a sexually transmitted infection; Act consistently with one's own values when dealing with an unintended pregnancy; Seek early prenatal care; Help prevent sexual abuse; Demonstrate respect for people with different sexual values; Exercise democratic responsibility to influence legislation dealing with sexual issues; Assess the impact of family, cultural, media and societal messages on one's thoughts, feelings, values and behaviours related to sexuality; Critically examine the world around them for biases based on gender, sexual orientation, culture, ethnicity and race; Promote the rights of all people to accurate sexuality information; Avoid behaviours that exhibit prejudice and bigotry; Reject stereotypes about the sexuality of different populations; Educate others about sexuality (adapted from Sexuality Information and Education Council of the United States 2004, pp. 16–17).
7 Both men and women have access to additional partners in polyamorous relationships, distinguishing them from polygamy.

## References

Besnier, N. and Alexeyeff, K., (eds), 2014. *Gender on the edge: Transgender, gay, and other Pacific Islanders*. Honolulu, HI: University of Hawai'i Press.

Blake, S. in conversation with Aggleton, P., 2016. Young people, sexuality and diversity. What does a needs-led and rights-based approach look like? *Sex Education*, 17 (3), 363–369. doi:10.1080/14681811.2016.1233015

Buck, P.H., 1939. *Anthropology and religion*. New Haven: Yale University Press.

Butler, J., 2004. *Undoing gender*. New York: Routledge.

Childs, P. and Williams, P., 2013. *Introduction to post-colonial theory*. New York: Routledge.

Cook Islands Ministry of Education, 2006. *Oraanga e te Tupuanga Meitaki: Health and physical wellbeing curriculum*. Rarotonga, Cook Islands: Ministry of Education.

Cook Islands Ministry of Finance and Economic Management, 2012. *Cook Islands 2011 Census of Population and Dwellings*. Rarotonga: Ministry of Finance and Economic Management.

Cook Islands Ministry of Finance and Economic Management, 2016. *Cook Islands Population Census 2016*. Rarotonga: Cook Islands Government.

Cook Islands Ministry of Health and Secretariat of the Pacific Community, 2007. *Second generation surveillance surveys of antenatal women and youth: Cook Islands 2005–2006*. Available from: https://www.aidsdatahub.org/resource/second-generation-surveillance-surveys-antenatal-women-and-youth-cook-islands-2005–2006

Cook Islands Ministry of Internal Affairs: Youth Suicide Prevention Steering Committee, 2015. *Rangi Marie: Youth Suicide Prevention Report to Government*. Rarotonga: Cook Islands Government.

Crocombe, R. and Holmes, R., 2014. *The impact of Europeans upon Southern Cook Islands Maori society, customary law and land tenure law 1595–1888 = Te Turanga o te Iti Tangata Maori i te Pa Enua Tonga o te Kuki Airani i muri ake i te taeanga mai o te papaa, e te au papa ture tupuna e te au papa ture enua 1595–1888*. Rarotonga: The Cook Islands Library and Museum Society Incorporated.

Davies, B., 2000. The concept of agency. In: *A body of writing, 1990–1999*. Walnut Creek, CA: AltaMira Press, 55–68.

Fine, M., 1988. Sexuality, schooling and adolescent females: The missing discourse of desire. *Harvard Educational Review*, 58 (1), 29–51. doi:10.17763/haer.58.1.u0468k1v2n2n8242

Futter-Puati, D., 2017a. *Api'ianga Tupuanga Kopapa: Sexuality Education in the Cook Islands*. PhD thesis. RMIT, Melbourne, Australia.

Futter-Puati, D., 2017b. Api'ianga Tupuanga Kopapa: Sexuality Education in the Cook Islands. Sexuality and Relationships Education, Years 9 and 10. Available from: https://researchrepository.rmit.edu.au/esploro/outputs/doctoral/Apiianga-tupuanga-kopapa-Sexuality-education-in-the-Cook-Islands/9921863878301341#file-1 [Accessed 25 November 2021].

Futter-Puati, D. and Maua-Hodges, T., 2019. Stitching tivaevae: a Cook Islands research method. *AlterNative: An International Journal of Indigenous Peoples*, 15 (2), 140–149. doi:10.1177/1177180119836788

Gilbert, J., 2014. *Sexuality in school: The limits of education*. Minneapolis: University of Minnesota Press.

Iyler, P. and Aggleton, P., 2015. Seventy years of sex education in *Health Education Journal*: A critical review. *Health Education*, 74 (1), 3–15. 10.1177/0017896914523942

Jackson, A.Y. and Mazzei, L.A., 2012. *Thinking with theory in qualitative research: Viewing data across multiple perspectives*. New York: Routledge.

Kelly-Hanku, A., et al., 2021. From the researched to the researcher: Decolonising research praxis in Papua New Guinea. In: S. Bell, P. Aggleton, and A. Gibson (eds), *Peer research in health and social development: International perspectives on participatory research*. Abingdon: Routledge, 22–32.

Ministry of Foreign Affairs and Trade, 2021. About Cook Islands. Available from: https://www.mfat.govt.nz/nl/countries-and-regions/australia-and-pacific/cook-islands/new-zealand-high-commission-to-the-cook-islands/about-cook-islands/ [Accessed 30 November 2021]

Naz, R., 2014. Sex education in Fiji. *Sexuality & Culture*, 18 (3), 664–687. doi:10.1007/s12119-013-9204-3

Ollis, D., 2015. 'I felt like i was watching porn': The reality of preparing pre-service teachers to teach about sexual pleasure. *Sex Education*, 16 (3), 308–323. doi:10.1080/14681811.2015.1075382

Radio New Zealand, 2012. Population explosion looms in the Pacific, parliamentarians warn. [Radio], 7 June. Retrieved from http://www.radionz.co.nz/international/pacific-news/205088/population-explosion-looms-in-pacific,-parliamentarians-warn [Accessed 16 November 2021]

Reeves, R., 2012. Small island states = large ocean states. *Cook Islands News*, 28 August. Available from: https://www.cookislandsnews.com/regional/small-island-states-large-ocean-states/ [Accessed 24 November 2021].

Secretariat of the Pacific Community, 2010. *Assessment report of adolescent sexuality education (or family life education) in ten PICTs*. Available from: https://web2.unfpa.org/public/about/oversight/evaluations/docDownload.unfpa?docId=105 [Accessed 30 Decmber 2021].

Sexuality Information and Education Council of the United States, 2004. *Guidelines for comprehensive sexuality education: Kindergarten through 12th grade*. 3rd ed. New York: Sexuality Information and Education Council of the United States.

Sheff, E., 2005. Polyamorous women, sexual subjectivity and power. *Journal of Contemporary Ethnography*, 34 (3), 251–283. doi:10.1177/0891241604274263

Smith, L. and Gunn, A., 2015. Challenging the pervasiveness of heteronormativity. In: A. Gunn and L. Smith (eds), *Sexual cultures in Aotearoa New Zealand education*. Dunedin: Otago University Press, 226–239.

Smith, L.T., 2012. *Decolonizing methodologies: Research and indigenous peoples*. 2nd ed. Dunedin, New Zealand: University of Otago Press.

Thammaraksa, P., et al., 2014. Helping teachers conduct sex education in secondary schools in Thailand: Overcoming culturally sensitive barriers to sex education. *Asian Nursing Research*, 8 (2), 99–104. doi:10.1016/j.anr.2014.04.001

Vai'imene, G., 2003. Api'i: Culture in education. In: R. Crocombe and M. Crocombe (eds), *Akono'anga Maori: Cook Islands culture*. Rarotonga: Institute of Pacific Studies and Cook Islands Extension Centre: University of the South Pacific in association with the Cook Islands Cultural and Historic Places Trust and the Ministry of Cultural Development, 169–178.

Varani-Norton, E., 2014. 'It's good to teach them, but … they should also know when to apply it': parents' views and attitudes towards Fiji's Family Life Education curriculum. *Sex Education*, 14 (6), 1–5. doi:10.1080/14681811.2014.934443

# 5 A Positive Youth Development approach to addressing sexual and gender diversity with Pasifika young people in Australia

*Jioji Ravulo*

## Introduction

Prior to colonisation and the work of missionaries in Oceania, Pacific-Indigenous communities practised diverse ways of knowing and doing, being and becoming, that continue to permeate views and values in contemporary societies today – both in the Pacific and in the Pacific diaspora. These include the embedded notion of egalitarianism, whereby everyone is valued and has a role to play in promoting the common good, harmony and well-being of all. However, not all traditional views remain, including the way in which diverse sexualities and genders, and accompanying norms, values and behaviours were previously seen as a source of strength and unity.

In this chapter, I use the terms and concept of Pacific, Pasifika and Pacific-Indigenous interchangeably. All the terms mean the same and may be used to represent the people of the Moana/Oceania/South Pacific region, including Melanesia, Micronesia, Polynesia and their diasporas locally, regionally and globally. As Pacific people we will individually and collectively decide how we will be 'labelled' and referenced within our own spaces, spaces which continue to be colonised by white and westerned views and values. This chapter explores the diverse forms of sexuality and gender that were practised before colonisation with the view to engaging with and embracing such differences today. A Positive Youth Development framework that supports a sociohistorical and sociocultural lens is advanced to promote ways to meaningfully support the well-being of Pasifika young people. Benefits to psychosocial development can result from the use of such an apporach, prompting supportive family dynamics, community engagement and social inclusion.

Talking openly about sexuality and gender diversity and accompanying practices can be challenging in modern Pacific family settings – especially within the context of conservative religious views and values. We have seen this play out in comments and actions made by Pacific elite athletes in Australia, including by Israel Folau which resulted in his high profile sacking by Rugby Australia, and the decision by six Manly Sea Eagles Rugby League players to not wear the club's inaguaral Pride jersey (Ravulo 2022). Understanding and upholding contemporary Pasifika gender and sexuality norms and expectations in

DOI: 10.4324/9781003142072-6

our communities reinforces these expectations and greatly influences the context in which people of diverse genders and sexuality can live and act. The shame and stigma that develops and is maintained by needing to uphold these conservative views and values are unhelpful and hinder approaches to developing a more progressive, open and respectful stance on sexuality and gender, as I have sought to do in my practice. But it was not always this way for many communities and cultures across the Pacific.

Before colonial influences, including the work of Christian missionaries, Pacific-Indigenous (also commonly known as Pasifika) genders and sexualities were fluid and organically driven by the desire to connect within community (Ravulo 2021). In many communities men would have sex with men without shame and stigma, as such practices were undertaken as a way of relating socially to others. Under the impact of colonisation, Christian teaching was used to condemn such practices, forcing judgement on such sexualised forms of behaviour. Sexuality and gender have long been and still are integral to promoting happy, healthy relationships with others, providing a platform for self-expression and a sacred space to be nurtured and nourished (Presterudstuen 2019). Across the Pacific, our physical and naked bodies were once seen as a source of strength and beauty, with cultural performances including dance providing a vehicle to share stories and narratives bound to special spaces and places. Such practices are still performed across ceremonies and special occasions including weddings and community gatherings. However, we were told to cover up and denounce such erotic forms of expressions in the context of civility and conformity.

In this chapter, I will embrace the value of sexuality and gender diversity in supporting the psychosocial development of Pacific-Indigenous young people. The context in which I engage with these issues is in questioning the hegemonic, dominant white and westernised expressions, views, labels and practices thrust upon modern Pacific communities both within countries of origin and in the Pacific diaspora globally. Much of my own work across fields of practices including youth offending, mental health literacy and harmful substance use has aimed to empower our young people to have a voice and to share their own lived experiences with the self and others in a safe space. This includes project-based work in Australia, Aotearoa New Zealand, Fiji, Tonga, Samoa and Vanuatu. The need to adopt a strengths-based approach in supporting young people to navigate and negotiate their evolving identities is crucial to creating prosocial attitudes and behaviours.

Responsibility for such approaches needs to be shared, however, with individuals seeing their role in the collective as part of the bigger picture in enabling families and communities to thrive. The need to ensure our social structures, systems and services operate to maintain this strength-based approach is imperative to achieving shared success. This is where diverse perspectives on psychosocial youth development, along with a Positive Youth Development framework, can be of benefit. A key perspective that helps shape my approach is the use of a sociohistorical lens. This provides an understanding of how unhelpful views about sexuality and gender within Pacific communities may have developed. A sociocultural lens also helps identify possible resources that practitioners – including youth workers, educators, health professionals and peers working alongside Pasifika young people – may use to develop a prosocial view of sexuality and gender. Previous tools I have used will be examined, along with a new programme that has been developed from my ongoing work in the community which employs a *talanoa* approach to social change.

It is my hope that through talanoa — shared conversation — with young people, their peers, parents, carers, educators, professional support people and the wider community we can meaningfully support Pasifika youth whilst enhancing their psychosocial development, civic engagement and overall well-being. The need to develop models of service delivery and provision that incorporate a whole of family practice approach is central to this engagement. To create positive change, it is essential for Pacific young people to be understood within the family, community and broader social context. We need to move beyond the pathologisation of individual problems commonly found in Western discourses, to more collective and collaborative perspectives that complement Pacific views and values.

## Exploring and embracing diverse sexualities and gender identities

Pasifika communities across the region have long celebrated gender and sexuality diversity within their social structures and systems (Elliston 1995; Murray 2002), embracing the need to support one another within a collective context (Neill 2009). Numerous concepts within our communities promote a communal approach, in which everyone is valued, and everyone plays their part in supporting a happy healthy community. Within iTaukei families, for example, values such as *solesolevaki* (reciprocal giving and living), *veiqaravi* (service to others), and *vakarokoroko* (reverent and respectful interactions) are promoted, whereby my well-being is your well-being, my resources are shared and I am valued as part of the community. Similar cultural concepts on the role of the collective, and the importance given to reciprocal living can be found in other communities across the Pacific.

A culture of acceptance is created through these shared values and views. As our societies are broadly egalitarian in nature, everyone has a role to play. Everyone is seen as part of the community, and a person's sense of belonging and individual identity is inextricably tied to others. Many Pasifika communities also strive to enact the notion of there being *vā* or *tabu* (sacred space) between the self and others, ensuring equilibrium is sought as part of creating a community in which everyone's well-being is supported in a shared and reciprocal way.

Our collective ability to express and adhere to these principles is challenged by the complex contexts we now traverse. A Pasifika diaspora can be found in many Western countries, including Australia, Aotearoa New Zealand, the United States of America, Japan, the UK and in other European countries. In all of these settings, we are challenged to compete with capitalist beliefs about society and what it means to participate on the global stage. Along with such expectations has come the need to assimilate individualistic ways of knowing and doing, being and becoming. The desire to consume, grow personal wealth and profit from our interactions with others has transformed Pacific people's sense of self and connection with others. Our views of the world experience pressure to change so as to align with Western knowledges and ideas, and the logic and 'science' that underpins them. As a result, Pasifika people now live within systems and structures that purport the existence of a binary – in the form of a right and wrong way of navigating the world. Our more fluid and organic ways of understanding and living are seen as outdated, outmoded, misplaced and mismatched in modern society. Church-based practices, including those promoted by Christianity, also create static and fixed ways of knowing and interacting with the world, with consequences for how we view sexuality and gender diversity.

Colonisation and its ongoing expression through neo-colonialism and neo-imperialism continues to play out across our Island and diasporic communities. Missionaries and the broader Christian movement across the Pacific region – sometimes led by Pacific Islanders themselves (Teauariki 1996) – impacted and displaced previous cultural perspectives by suggesting that many traditional practices were evil and anti-monotheistic. Pacific people have been conditioned to reject our previous views on sexuality, including diverse sexualities and genders, and have been told that these were wrong. As a result, our own Lesbian, Gay, Bisexual, Transgender, Intersex, Queer, Asexual and other sexually or gender diverse (LGBTIQA+) community members are seen as outsiders, with legislation still in place in various Pacific Islands states and territories to criminalise their behaviour. The majority of our Pacific Islands, including the Cook Islands, Kiribati, Papua New Guinea, Samoa, Solomon Islands, Tonga and Tuvalu retain laws criminalising homosexuality. Despite Fiji lifting such punitive laws in 2010, widespread discrimination still takes place. The legacies of colonialism and missionisation remain strong.

However, there is hope. Queer Pacific people and their allies are breaking through in contemporary settings, reclaiming traditional views and values with the desire to transform Pacific discourses and narratives. Advocacy, support and lobby groups run by Pasifika for Pasifika in Australia, Aotearoa New Zealand and the broader Oceania region are leading this movement. They include the Pacific Sexual and Gender Diversity Network (PSGDN 2022) that strives to mobilise, mediate, advocate, strengthen and celebrate Queer Pacific people and their inclusion across the Pacific Islands and our diaspora globally. Social media is used to share stories of resilience and resistance. PSGDN has also created and moderate a private group called LGBT Pacific with over 1,000 members to assist in creating a safe space in which to critically review and discuss matters affecting LGBTIQA+ people in the Pacific region.

In support of all of our youth, there is an ongoing need to explore and embrace Pasifika ways of knowing and doing, being and becoming, before colonisation, Christianity, capitalism and consumerism. This includes engaging with how we previously perceived and practised diverse genders and sexualities.

It also includes reclaiming key concepts such *solesolevaki*, *veiqaravi*, *vakarokoroko*, *vā* and *tabu*. As Pacific-Indigenous cultures are relationally driven and focussed, we can utilise cultural practices like talanoa to help drive and shape our views and values. A talanoa approach provides opportunities for individuals to come together, to be part of a communal conversation that is shaped by the lived experiences of others, and to move forward, together. A talanoa approach offers an organic and fluid process in which people can feel safe to explore and embrace their sense of self within a supportive context. And it is through such practices that we can learn the value of reciprocity, service, respect and sacred space irrespective of sexuality or gender.

## Promoting diversity through Positive Youth Development

I turn now to explore an approach called Positive Youth Development, with a view to understanding its potential to promote diversity. The approach described relates to work I have undertaken with adolescents and strives to support the young person's development in a broader context as they move towards adulthood.

Western psychology and philosophies have paved the way for life course perspectives (or a focus on lifespan development) to be researched and written about. Many scholars have anchored their ontology, epistemology and axiology within an individualistic framework, whereby the person is individually seen for their ability to function and contribute to society and its shared values and purposes. Adolescence, which in Western contexts is generally understood as happening between the ages of 12 and 24, but in the Pacific youth can be up to 35 years, is seen as the gateway to a becoming a functional adult. It is argued that failure to successfully navigate and negotiate adolescence can lead to problematic interpersonal and intrapersonal social skills that have a later impact on a person's ability to function as a member of society. This includes their ability to engage in educational and employment opportunities, intimate relationships and health literacies. In line with such notions, responsibility is generally placed on the individual to fit in, and to shape their behaviour in accordance with social norms and values. It is often assumed individuals will undertake a linear path of progression during this time, to emerge with valuable insights, understanding and a sense of purpose in life.

For young people, whatever we call this stage of life, it is a point of transition. Children are physically transformed from their childlike state. They become more aware of a sense of self physically, mentally, spiritually, ethically and economically. They may also start to see themselves as sexual beings, gradually becoming more aware of what they are attracted to and who they attract. Their perspectives on what constitutes their gender identity are expressed through their interactions with the self and others. Their ability to explore physical and sexual intimacy will be shaped by their understanding of what is perceived to be acceptable within the status quo.

If the status quo insists that your sexuality and gender expression is rigidly in line with the moralities imposed by others, then many young people will be left feeling undesirable and mismatched. This can greatly challenge a positive sense of self-worth, self-value, self-esteem and self-love. Negative or maladaptive processes ensue and may become entrenched in someone's burgeoning identity, leading to problematic and unhelpful feelings and behaviours. Such attributes are then carried through into adulthood, where they continue to play out across social interactions. The individual is left to their own devices and, as a result, society produces groups that struggle with fitting in. Limited accountability is placed on social structures and systems, views and values that perpetuate these outcomes.

### *Positive Youth Development and its prosocial impacts*

As one way of engaging with these issues, Positive Youth Development strives to engage with broader social and systemic factors in a more meaningful way when supporting young people through adolescent development. Founded on an ecological perspective and developmental systems theories (Silbereisen and Lerner 2012), the framework is underpinned by understanding the vast number of variables that may impact on the individual and their development (Arnold 2017). Rather than placing exclusive responsibility on the person, this perspective recognises and holds to account the impact of social structures and systems that may create problems (Seymour 2017). At the same time, it identifies opportunities to reshape narratives so as to be more inclusive of diversity, whilst prompting change to occur from this point of difference (Sherrod 2007). For example, if a young person is finding it difficult to engage within an education setting, responsibility is placed on such learning environments to naturally evolve and change in their ability to fit and respond to diverse needs. Overall, Positive Youth Development strives to reframe adolescence as a positive process, rather than one of deficit. It works with the whole person in their broader context(s) and utilises knowledge in shaping journeys that are characterised by resilience and hope.

There are two key hypotheses and a series of sub-hypotheses within a Positive Youth Development approach, as outlined by Silbereisen and Lerner (2012, pp. 5–7):

1 Youth-context alignment promotes Positive Youth Development

- Provides scope for a young person's strengths to a be a key focus and respectively aligned to resources made available for their development
  - Contextual alignment involves marshalling development assets
- Adequate resources (e.g. education, health) are aligned in promoting strengths
  - Community-based programmes are a vital source of developmental assets
- Programmes are designed and funded to ensure a proactive process of support if provided to young people and their positive development

2 Positive Youth Development is composed of five Cs

- Competence, confidence, connection, character and caring
  - Contribution is the 'sixth C'
- Provoking civic participation to occur as a result
  - Positive Youth Development and risk/problem behaviours are inversely related
- Issues are mitigated as a result of creating and implementing a Positive Youth Development approach

Programmes based on a Positive Youth Development framework enable individual lived experiences to become part of a broader collective understanding shared by adolescents (Arahanga-Doyle et al. 2019). A Positive Youth Development-informed programme values the diverse perspectives of its participants and encourages these voices to shape outputs and outcomes (Fredricks and Simpkins 2012). As a way of working with young people, Positive Youth Development has evolved over many decades and continues to be a driving force in youth development programmes globally (Arnold 2017). Due to its organic nature, it offers an ideal framework for working with cultural diversity and its differences (Kenyon and Hanson 2012).

## Promoting Positive Youth Development with Pasifika young people

I joined the social work profession with a passion to work alongside young people, especially those considered to be on the margins of society. My first full-time job was working as a post release support caseworker – assisting young people who offend to reintegrate into their communities after spending time in custody. I was based in greater western Sydney, where one of Australia's largest urbanised populations of Pasifika people live; as a result, a large proportion of my case load were Pasifika young people. As my role expanded, so did my responsibility to oversee and create developmental programmes that were culturally nuanced and safe for our Pacific families (Ravulo 2016). One of the key challenges in working with Pacific young people who offend lay in understanding their health literacies, and how these played out across their lives. Access to resources alongside health responses within the family differed, with a major reliance on parental knowledges and perspectives.

A series of group-based workshops was created under key areas of need. Fondly titled 'In Da Know,' each workshop was created to be an interactive and engaging dialogically driven process across five true or false questions (Ravulo and Mission Australia 2009). Three of the five In Da Know workshops were related to health: In Da Know Mental Health, In Da Know Alcohol and Other Drugs, and In Da Know Sexual Health. These workshops were designed to be delivered by a single facilitator and were open to groups of young Pasifika people who had already offended, were deemed at risk of offending, and at high school. Each group was facilitated based on geographical areas in which the young person lived or was enrolled and might include all three groups of youth.

Within the In Da Know Sexual Health Quick Questionnaire, five true or false questions were used as a basis for talanoa:

1 You can't get AIDS by having vaginal sex
2 If a girl uses the 'Pill' then she is protected against sexually transmitted infections
3 Most common sexually transmitted infections can be cured (if something is done as soon as possible!)
4 You can always physically tell that you have a sexually transmitted infection
5 There is no place I can go to speak about my sexual health

Due to the sensitive nature of the workshop content, activities generally took place in separate groups of male and female participants. A facilitator's guide was provided, overviewing answers to each question along with the rationale along with further details to support a shared conversation. The facilitators included myself and fellow case workers employed by a community-based programme I was leading at the time. Additional resources were also signposted to support each answer, ranging from community-based health services to websites. A banana-shaped penis was used for condom demonstration in these workshops, providing Pasifika young people with an opportunity to talk about safe sex practices and other issues.

Responses from Pasifika young people who participated in this workshop were generally positive. Feedback was obtained through worksheets provided to young people at each session. A supportive and safe space that privileged the views and voice of young people was created by ensuring every participant was provided with an opportunity to share their views on the themes being discussed. The setting provided scope for young people to raise and explore other related questions, including their varying views on maintaining perceived virginity by valuing and having oral or anal rather than vaginal sex, how to access resources without parents knowing, and how to be a supportive friend. Such youth initiated and led content enabled Pasifika young people to talk candidly about their experiences whilst reframing their sexuality and gender as a helpful part of their identity.

The above approach and the implementation of In Da Know workshops strongly resonated with the Positive Youth Development framework. The programme focused heavily on the contributions of young Pasifika people – with each of the five true or false questions based on the experiences they had with their sexual health, gleaned from my previous work with Pacific-Indigenous young people, and the trends I encountered in my casework with them. The need to create the series of workshops came from a lack of nuanced programmes for Pasifika young people in Australia, and my desire to ensure that new resources were created and properly aligned. The sexual health content within the workshop was tailored to include the voice of Pacific young people and their broader capabilities to navigate and negotiate these areas of their well-being. The workshops prompted competencies to be developed in health literacy, in turn provoking confidence, a connection to each other and to accessing further support if needed. Implementing such programmes promoted individual and collective help-seeking behaviour, whilst promoting a level of self-care for self and others. Civic responsibility may also develop by empowering young people to engage in prosocial behaviours and counteracting risky problematic perspectives and practices.

Aligning this work to a Positive Youth Development framework offered service providers the opportunity to consider the sociohistorical and sociocultural contexts in which Pacific young people and their families are located. It challenged the status quo by providing health services to consumers based on their own terms, rather than the terms of structures and systems that are designed to make people 'fit in.'

## Healthy relationships talanoa: Understanding the role of sexuality and gender with Pasifika youth

With Positive Youth Development in mind, I want to outline a new programme to further support youth development. This time the focus is on exploring and embracing diverse sexualities and genders within Pasifika communities. This new programme strives to be dialogically driven and aims to support an initial and ongoing talanoa around healthy and respectful relationships. Aptly titled *Healthy Relationships Talanoa*, the programme encourages a shared approach to well-being. The themes underlying the questions explored include understanding sexuality and gender from a Pacific-Indigenous perspective. The conversations are shaped by the lived experience of the participants and enable facilitators to share something of the sociohistorical and sociocultural contexts in which sexuality and gender diversity may play out – from the past, present and future. As the group process is guided by a talanoa approach, it provides all participants with the opportunity to actively engage with the concepts being discussed.

This new programme was established alongside my current and ongoing work with community agencies working with Pacific young people in Western Sydney. In 2018, after the tragic passing of two young Pacific men by suicide (not related to issues of gender or sexuality), I helped establish a weekly *Wellbeing Talanoa* with young people in Bankstown in Western Sydney during the initial period of trauma/grief. As a result of this talanoa, the model was developed further and is now being utilised by Pacific youth workers, counsellors and social workers in various youth services and agencies across western Sydney to offer a shared and safe space for young people to talk about an array of issues, including mental health, educational and vocational aspirations, family dynamics, community, and cultural commitments. The creation of the *Healthy Relationships Talanoa* complements the existing suite of services offered across the community, and is being implemented through this network of professionals and local Pacific young people.

### *Healthy Relationship Talanoa (HRT) programme overview*

Like its earlier counterpart In Da Know, the HRT (pronounced *her-are-t*, like *heart*) programme seeks to privilege the perspectives of Pasifika young people, and their lived experiences. It supports the sharing of what may be known, unknown, explored and unpacked when embracing diverse sexualities and gender identities. In preparation to facilitate HRT, it is strongly recommended that facilitators access and read articles by Presterudstuen (2019), Redman-MacLaren and Veukiso-Ulugia (2019) and Ravulo (2021) to support their understanding of key concerns and relevant sociohistorical and sociocultural issues.

Each week, a specific question is raised to provide a platform for reflection in the hour-long talanoa. The physical room is set up with chairs forming a circle to encourage conversation. If the talanoa is hosted virtually (as some have had to be within the context of COVID-19), then participants are encouraged to have their videos switched on and share their audio when contributing. The facilitator works collaboratively to ensure a safe space is created. This includes reminding participants that the shared conversation is confidential and people are encouraged to share only how much they feel comfortable with. Other key group rules include ensuring people can share their views without shame and judgement, highlighting that respect for each other reigns.

Organically driven, each week the facilitator will ask each participant to introduce themselves via the following three 'check in' questions: name, Pasifika heritage, and how are you feeling today? This provides everyone with an opportunity to affirm and feel value for their Pacific identity and heritage, establishing that this is an integral part of the process and sharing space. The question about feelings is asked to help the facilitator understand how each person may be positioned emotionally, with the view that the same question will be asked again at the end of the group.

Throughout the talanoa, it is important that the facilitator uses inclusive language and an approach that is strengths-based and solution focussed. Deficits can be explored in the conversation, for example, negative views or perspectives that may impact on how people feel. Doing this is welcomed as part of the process of creating a shared conversation about ways to possibly challenge and counteract these negative views so as to move forward. An emphasis on challenging any unhelpful binaries including between male and female, and gay or straight is an important feature of the talanoa, ensuring people can share their views and values without fear of judgement or ridicule. The focus is on helpful perspectives that can shape healthy relationships.

After the introductions have taken place, the facilitator explores one of the four weekly reflection questions suggested below. Each person is asked to provide their feedback on the question, and the facilitator builds on what each person shares, to explore related themes and perspectives. As it is driven by a talanoa, the conversation can go anywhere, with the facilitator using this time to help participants safely make meaning of what is being discussed.

**Box 5.1 HRT weekly reflection questions**

1 *What does it mean to see the world through our own gender identity?*
This question strives to understand the diverse ways in which gender identity can mould and shape our values and how they play out across Pacific spaces, with a view to encouraging a broader understanding of how Pasifika people viewed such expectations and practices prior to colonisation.

2 *What has sexuality got to do with it?*
Who we are attracted to and who we attract has an impact on our sense of self and our broader identity. This topic will explore the way our sexuality is understood and how we can have a healthy relationship with it alongside other contexts, including faith and family.

3 *What does a healthy relationship look like?*
Intimate relationships are very rewarding and can provide many benefits to our well-being. Understanding the role we play in creating such safe relationships will be the focus of this conversation, exploring and embracing helpful ways to connect in varying ways.

4 *What does sex got to do with it?*
Promoting an understanding and developing insight into the role of our own sexualised behaviour is key to establishing happy, healthy relationships. This question provides participants with an opportunity to discuss safe sex practice, how to access helpful resources, and how to develop shareable knowledge and information on healthy approaches to sexual health overall.

As the talanoa is drawing to a close, the facilitator asks participants to 'check out' by each answering the following two questions: how are you feeling on the back of today's shared conversation; and what are the possible takeaways from our shared conversation? These questions are designed to assist facilitators to consolidate the key ideas shared from the talanoa, whilst ensuring individuals are expressing helpful feelings in association with their participation and broader engagement. Asking them also provides an opportunity to participants to come back the week after and access any additional support or resources needed. Of course, it is possible to develop other questions related to sexuality and gender diversity with Pacific-Indigenous communities with a view to identifying issues that a future talanoa might explore.

### *Reflecting a Positive Youth Development framework*

The *Healthy Relationship Talanoa* programme resonates strongly with the Positive Youth Development Framework through its approach which centres the contributions of Pasifika participants. It harnesses the diverse perspectives that people may bring to the conversation, whilst striving to understand what other structures may be at play within their interactions in this topic area. These include the influence of family, health care providers, educational environments, religious beliefs, welfare and legal knowledge. It empowers young people to be equipped with information on ways to understand themselves and how this contributes to their engagement with others. Competence, confidence, connection, character and caring are mobilised as Pasifika young people are learning to value their bodies, their own sense of sexuality and how this can translate to happy, healthy relationships.

## Concluding thoughts

As a social work practitioner, I am constantly inspired and motivated by opportunities to create space for Pacific-Indigenous perspectives to play out across society – whether it be within our own communities, in the diaspora, or in the homes of our heritage. I believe it is possible to include and meaningfully utilise traditional knowledges from the past in the present and into our futures. People who work alongside Pasifika communities are encouraged to shape their practices to be intentionally inclusive so young people are afforded the opportunity to shape the talanoa | conversations in which they participate. Through this, Pacific young people are afforded a voice and a platform on which to make informed decisions on important matters relevant their health and well-being. This can later translate to other forms of prosocial behaviours and attitudes that are shaped by a collectivist context that esteems diversity as the norm. It is through this shared approach that we can truly aspire towards an inclusive society that embraces sexuality and gender diversity in all communities.

## References

Arahanga-Doyle, H., et al., 2019. Positive Youth Development in Māori and New Zealand European adolescents through an adventure education programme. *Kotuitui*, 14 (1), 38–51. doi:10.1080/1177083X.2018.1508479

Arnold, M.E., 2017. Supporting adolescent exploration and commitment: Identity formation, thriving, and positive youth development. *Journal of Youth Development*, 12 (4), 1–15. doi:10.5195/JYD.2017.522

Elliston, D.A., 1995. Erotic anthropology: ritualized homosexuality in Melanesia and beyond. *American Ethnologist*, 22 (4), 848–867.

Fredricks, J.A. and Simpkins, S.D., 2012. Promoting positive youth development through organized after-school activities: Taking a closer look at participation of ethnic minority youth. *Child Development Perspectives*, 6 (3), 280–287. doi:10.1111/j.1750-8606.2011.00206.x

Kenyon, D.B. and Hanson, J.D., 2012. Incorporating traditional culture into positive youth development programs with American Indian/Alaska Native youth. *Child Development Perspectives*, 6 (3), 272–279. doi:10.1111/j.1750-8606.2011.00227.x

Murray, S.O., 2002. *Pacific homosexualities*. Lincoln, NE: Writers Club Press.

Neill, J., 2009. *The origins and role of same-sex relations in human societies*. Jefferson, NC: McFarland & Company.

Presterudstuen, G.H., 2019. Understanding sexual and gender diversity in the Pacific Islands. In: J. Ravulo, T. Mafile'o, and D.B. Yeates (eds), *Pacific social work: Navigating practice, policy and research*. Abingdon/New York: Routledge, 161–171.

PSGDN, 2022. [Facebook]. Available from: https://www.facebook.com/PSGDN [Accessed 3 August 2022]

Ravulo, J., 2016. An integrated case management model to assist pacific youth offenders and their families in Australia. *Care Management Journals*, 17 (4), 170–179. doi:10.1891/1521-0987.17.4.170

Ravulo, J., 2021. Exploring the role of sexuality and identity across the Pacific. In: H.N. Weaver (ed), *The Routledge international handbook of Indigenous resilience*. Abingdon/New York: Routledge, 108–120. doi:10.4324/9781003048428-10

Ravulo, J., 2022. Don't blame Pacific Island cultures for queer fear. Blame colonisation. *The Sydney Morning Herald*, 27 July. Avaialble from: https://www.smh.com.au/sport/don-t-blame-pacific-island-cultures-for-queer-fear-blame-colonisation-20220727-p5b50c.html [Accessed 3 August 2022].

Ravulo, J. and Mission Australia, 2009. *Developing and implementing a case management model for young people with complex needs: A toolkit for community workers, educators and justice officers*. Available from: https://nla.gov.au/nla.obj-254917404/view [Accessed 3 August 2022].

Redman-MacLaren, M. and Veukiso-Ulugia, A., 2019. An introduction to sexual and reproductive health and wellbeing for Pacific social work. In: J. Ravulo, T. Mafile'o, and D.B. Yeates (eds), *Pacific social work: navigating practice, policy and research*. Abingdon/New York: Routledge, 125–138.

Seymour, K., 2017. Building on strengths: A new framework for Positive Youth Development program practice. *Queensland Review*, 24 (1), 5–22. doi:10.1017/qre.2017.3

Sherrod, L., 2007. Civic engagement as an expression of Positive Youth Development. In: R.K. Silbereisen and R.M. Lerner (eds), *Approaches to Positive Youth Development*. London: SAGE, 59–74.

Silbereisen, R.K. and Lerner, R.M., 2012. Approaches to Positive Youth Development: A view of the issues. In: R.K. Silbereisen and R.M. Lerner (eds), *Approaches to positive youth development*. London: SAGE, 3–30.

Teauariki, T., 1996. *Mission to Papua: A Cook Islands missionary in Papua New Guinea 1963-1975*. University of the South Pacific Cook Islands Extension Centre, (ed). Rarotonga: USP Centre.

## Part II

# Sexual and reproductive health and well-being

# 6 Sexual and reproductive health needs, challenges and opportunities in the Pacific

*Alyce N. Wilson, Elissa C. Kennedy, Amanda Noovao Hill, Lisa M. Vallely, Pinip Wapi, Errollyn Tungunaboe, Meredith Tutumang and Alec Ekeroma*

## Introduction

Entrenched in sociocultural norms, taboos and practices, sexual and reproductive health needs are complex in the Pacific Islands region. Geographically dispersed populations, shortages of health care workers, restrictive laws, gender inequality, women and girls' lack of sexual autonomy, and poverty intersect, creating significant barriers to providing or accessing sexual and reproductive health services. In this context, many countries in the region report high levels of unmet need for contraception and unintended pregnancy, poor maternal and newborn health outcomes and high rates of sexually transmitted infections.

## Sociocultural determinants of sexual and reproductive health

For many people in the Pacific, discourse around sex, sexuality, reproduction and family occur through largely Christian moral frameworks (Kelly et al. 2010). For girls and women, importance is placed on virginity, and shame is associated with any deviation from this expectation. This causes women to discuss or explore sexuality in secret, with implications for seeking health care and the uptake of services such as contraception. In contrast, pre- or extramarital sex is seen as normal for boys and men, whose masculinity is linked to sexual conquest and experience, even if this appears to conflict with moral teaching about sex. These norms and values are embedded in traditional structures and cultures, with some research indicating that disapproval of premarital sex was present prior to colonisation and/or the introduction of Christianity (Kelly et al. 2010). These norms and values are also reinforced by traditional culture – *kastom* – principles or rules that govern everyday life, including matters related to gender, marriage, sexuality and sexual and reproductive health (Buchanan-Aruwafu 2007). In Vanuatu, for example, young people describe kastom as preventing discussion of sex and sexual and reproductive health between relatives, preventing unmarried people's access to sexual and reproductive health services and defining gender roles and norms that assign greater power and agency within intimate relationships to men

DOI: 10.4324/9781003142072-8

compared with women. Moral frameworks also strongly enforce heteronormativity, contributing to the stigma and discrimination experienced by transgender and gender and sexually diverse people. Restrictive cultural attitudes and norms, often re-enforced by outdated criminal laws, have heightened significance for young people, who as part of normal human development are exploring their sexuality, consolidating their gender identities and forming their first sexual, romantic and other types of relationships. As such, young people in the Pacific experience a disproportionality high burden of poor sexual and reproductive health compared with older adults (UNFPA 2021).

Gender differences in acceptance of premarital sex means unmarried girls in particular experience substantial stigma and discrimination for seeking sexual and reproductive health information or services, or worse, experiencing unintended pregnancy (Kennedy et al. 2013a). Gender norms also affect girls' and women's agency to negotiate or initiate discussion around sex, condoms and contraception with intimate partners, and their ability to refuse unwanted sex (Mitchell and Bennett 2020). In Vanuatu, both girls and boys describe girls' lack of power to negotiate safe sex as a contributor to unwanted pregnancy, and while girls more often describe being forced or coerced into unwanted sex, boys also experience substantial pressure from peers and older men to 'prove' their masculinity through sexual conquest, including the use of sexual violence (Kennedy et al. 2013a). Rigid gender norms also contribute to high rates of gender-based violence, which in turn contributes to poor sexual and reproductive health. Among ever-partnered Pacific women aged 15–24 years, 55% have ever experienced physical and/or sexual violence from a partner, and 5% have experienced sexual violence from a non-intimate partner (UNFPA 2021).

Harmful norms, attitudes and taboos also extend to providers of sexual and reproductive health services. Judgemental attitudes from health providers, and lack of privacy and confidentiality, are major contributors to poor access and quality of care (Mitchell and Bell 2020). Young people in Vanuatu, for example, report being shamed by health workers for seeking condoms or contraception, scolded for being sexually active before marriage and denied counselling or care (Kennedy et al. 2013b). Many health workers in Vanuatu continue to find it difficult to provide sexual and reproductive health services, particularly for unmarried young people, due to conflicts with their own beliefs or fear of community repercussions, despite recent efforts to improve health worker training in this regard (Kennedy et al. 2013b).

## Contraception, unintended pregnancy and unsafe abortion

Contraceptive use in the Pacific is low compared with other low- and middle-income countries, with approximately half of all Pacific women (married and unmarried sexually active women) who want to avoid pregnancy currently using a modern method (Dawson et al. 2021). While communities generally have positive attitudes towards family planning and contraception, particularly to support healthy families, this has not translated into widespread use (Gupta et al. 2020).

Many factors contribute to low contraceptive use in the Pacific. Limited access to sexual and reproductive health services and disrupted commodity supply (particularly for shorter-acting contraceptives) are notable barriers, most markedly for communities in geographically remote locations (Dawson et al. 2021). Knowledge of contraception, including awareness of different methods, is also limited and misconceptions about reproduction and pregnancy, such as the belief that pregnancy is not possible during first sex, also contribute to low use (Cammock et al. 2018). Myths and misconceptions regarding modern contraception side effects or longer-term impacts are also common. In Tonga, for example, women have described beliefs that injectables and implants cause tiredness or backpain, and how the intrauterine device can become lost in the reproductive tract (Winn-Dix et al. 2016). Other health problems (such as neck pain) are also commonly attributed to contraceptive use (Winn-Dix et al. 2016). Similar misconceptions have been noted in Vanuatu and Papua New Guinea, including beliefs that some contraceptives cause cancer, weakness and infertility (Kennedy et al. 2014; Gupta et al. 2020). This misinformation or hearsay within communities has been reported to discourage use or contribute to discontinuation of contraception. While improved access to reliable health information about contraceptives is critical, so too is understanding of contraceptive use and preferences in the social and cultural context. In Papua New Guinea, for example, information about modern contraceptives provided by healthcare workers was considered trustworthy if it could be validated and corroborated with social and religious information concerning family planning, obtained through discussion with relatives, friends and respected community leaders (Gupta et al. 2020).

Cultural norms and religious beliefs are critical to understanding patterns of use, non-use and discontinued use of contraception. The importance of family and status associated with parenthood contributes to low use and, in some settings, lower demand for contraception. However, even where there are cultural expectations that promote fertility, a significant proportion of women, and men, report wanting to delay, space or limit their family size for health and/or economic reasons (Gilbert et al. 2016). Religious beliefs (particularly Christian beliefs) are an important influence on contraceptive use and acceptance in the Pacific, with children described as a 'blessing from God' and therefore the use of contraception is considered forbidden (Gilbert et al. 2016).While there may be an acceptance of traditional methods of family planning for married couples - to limit family size for example — there remains strong disapproval of use of modern methods, particularly by unmarried women and girls, and the belief that this leads to promiscuity.

In the Solomon Islands, religious leaders have been reported to directly intervene to discourage people from using contraception or preventing access to sexual and reproductive health clinics that provided such services (Gilbert et al. 2016). Cultural taboos and religious beliefs also contribute to the stigma or shame experienced by people seeking contraceptive services, and embarrassment or reluctance to access contraceptive methods, such as the intrauterine device, that require pelvic examination (Winn-Dix et al. 2016). Additionally, people living with disability and those with diverse forms of sexual orientation or gender identity/expression experience substantial unmet need for sensitive and responsive counselling and services relating to contraception. Lack of data and qualitative studies describing their experiences and needs contributes to their sexual and reproductive health needs being largely invisible in the Pacific region (UNFPA 2021).

Despite being considered 'women's business,' men have a strong influence over women's use of contraception and choice of method, with positive male involvement associated with women's increased use of modern contraceptive (Peach et al. 2021). Due to gender norms, women have less agency to initiate or negotiate contraceptive use. This is particularly true in the context of physical and/or sexual violence, In Fiji, for example, it was found that 10% of women who had experienced violence reported that their partner had refused or stopped contraception (Fiji Women's Crisis Centre 2013). Partner disapproval or objection is a common reason for women's unmet need for contraception, related to men's cultural or religious objections, reproductive control and desire to have more children (and/or sons), fear of side effects for their partner (such as weight gain or infertility), fear of side effects for themselves (such as the belief that a woman's use of injectables could cause weakness in their partner) and dislike of methods such as condoms because of concerns that they reduce sexual pleasure (Imtishal and Mohammadnezhad 2021). In Papua New Guinea, women report using methods such as intrauterine devices or injectables to overcome possible partner objection (Gupta et al. 2020).

There are many barriers to men being more positively engaged in contraceptive services, including limited contraceptive choices for men beyond male condoms and vasectomy, lack of information targeting men and limited access to sexual and reproductive health services that are welcoming or inclusive of men. Taboos discussing sex and contraception with opposite sex health providers and lack of good quality contraceptive counselling that includes men and/or couples are other notable barriers (Imtishal and Mohammadnezhad 2021). As such, many women and couples may not use any method to prevent unwanted pregnancy, or rely on less effective methods such as withdrawal or traditional methods.

In a context of high unmet contraceptive need, unintended pregnancy is common in many Pacific countries (see Tu'i'onetoa et al., Chapter 10), with available estimates indicating that up to 46% of pregnancies in the region are unintended, of which around 44% end in an induced abortion (Sully et al. 2019). Consequences of unintended pregnancy can be substantial for unmarried girls. Girls in Vanuatu and the Cook Islands describe fear, guilt and in some cases family violence as the result of unintended pregnancy, and many consider or seek abortion (McMillan and Worth 2011; White et al. 2018). Reflecting cultural and Christian beliefs that strongly condemn termination of a pregnancy, induced abortion, even on medical grounds, remains highly legally restricted in many countries. Even where abortion is legally permitted, access is constrained with women not able to access services due to the stigma associated with induced abortion and health care workers' refusal, often on religious grounds, to perform the service. As a result, many women turn to alternative, often unsafe, methods. Such methods include traditional and herbal abortifacients and physical and mechanical methods such as squeezing or tying ropes around the abdomen and undertaking excessive physical activity and drinking excessive amounts of instant coffee (Vallely et al. 2015). Off market use of misoprostol – a drug used widely in obstetrics and gynaecology — has also been described by women (Vallely et al. 2015).

Reasons for terminating a pregnancy include wanting to continue education studies, relationship issues, financial concerns and other socio-cultural factors, such as bringing shame or embarrassment to their families for being pregnant whilst unmarried or a student. In many countries in the Pacific being pregnant while receiving an education either at high school or at a university can result in a girl's expulsion, further disadvantaging them. Young iTaukei (Indigenous) Fijian women have described experiences of sexual and reproductive coercion, where male partners would coerce women into having an unwanted abortion (Mitchell and Bennett 2020). Tactics used by male partners included denial of paternity, refusal to support the mother and child, threatened violence and accusations of infidelity. However, occasions when male partners would discourage and prevent a woman from having a wanted abortion were also described.

## Maternal health and well-being

Across the Pacific, bearing children is a role of fundamental importance, not just for individuals and their families but for entire communities. In Tonga, for example, women have described the honour associated with motherhood and the honour afforded to mothers by the community, as well as the importance of motherhood to their lives and social status (Reed et al. 2017). However, for many women and their babies, pregnancy and childbirth are also times of risk. Despite global improvements in maternal mortality, many Pacific Island countries continue to experience unacceptably high rates of maternal death, and complications of pregnancy and childbirth remain a leading cause of death of girls aged 15–19 years (Institute for Health Metrics and Evaluation 2017). For example, in Papua New Guinea, official estimates of maternal mortality range from 170 to 730 deaths per 100,000 live births (Robbers et al. 2019). Real rates are likely to be even higher, as in Papua New Guinea and across the Pacific many women give birth at home or in the community and are therefore not counted. In addition, high rates of preterm birth, perinatal loss and newborn mortality are also reported in many Pacific Island countries.

Within the region, a number of factors contribute to poor maternal and newborn health including sexually transmitted infections, poor nutrition and iron-deficiency anaemia, malaria and other infectious diseases and, increasingly, non-communicable diseases, adolescent pregnancy, unsafe abortion and gender-based violence (Wilson et al. 2020). A key driver of poor health outcomes is limited access to good quality care during pregnancy and childbirth. Despite women and men having awareness of the complications that can arise during childbirth and the importance of antenatal care and supervised birth, regular care during pregnancy and childbirth is unavailable in many settings, most markedly in Papua New Guinea, where only 54% of women receive at least one antenatal visit from a health worker and only 40% give birth in a facility (National Department of Health 2019). For women living in rural or remote communities there may be financial, geographical and logistical barriers to reaching health services, particularly time-sensitive care during labour (Vallely et al. 2015).

Limited access to facilities that provide basic or comprehensive emergency obstetric care, under-resourced facilities with lack of equipment and other supplies, and significant health worker shortages contribute to challenges providing quality care (Wilson et al. 2020). Also lacking is access to respectful maternity care, defined as care that maintains dignity, privacy and confidentiality, ensures freedom from harm and mistreatment and enables informed choice and continuous support during labour and childbirth. Many women in the Pacific describe experiencing disrespectful or judgemental care during pregnancy and childbirth. Women in Papua New Guinea, for example, report fear of being scolded or shamed by providers, and rude or unfriendly care as deterrents to giving birth in a health facility (Vallely et al. 2015). Similarly, women in Samoa describe shame for not understanding medical jargon, lack of providers' recognition or respect for their own expert knowledge about childbirth and child health, and power imbalances with providers contributing to negative experiences in health care settings (Pio and Nosa 2020).

Customary and cultural factors also have a significant impact on the health and well-being of women during pregnancy, childbirth and the postnatal period. Many customary beliefs and practices are protective. In Tonga, for example, the extended family plays a significant role in providing support to new mothers through health advice, food preparation and care for other children (Reed et al. 2017). Female relatives in many countries have a direct role to play in supporting women during labour and acting as 'gatekeepers' to ensure new mothers have adequate rest and privacy during the postpartum period (Vallely et al. 2015). Similarly, taboos during pregnancy, such as avoiding excessive physical exertion or eating healthy food, may be beneficial to the health of women during pregnancy. However, other customary practices and taboos may contribute to lack of health care-seeking during pregnancy or birth. In Tonga, for example, women describe the importance and cultural significance of having a vaginal birth without medical intervention and how the stigma associated with assisted birth may deter care-seeking (Reed et al. 2017). In Papua New Guinea, cultural beliefs about menstrual or postpartum blood causing sickness, and taboos about being seen during birth (especially by men), contribute to women giving birth in seclusion or secret, remaining in birthing huts until postpartum bleeding has stopped (Vallely et al. 2015). Beliefs about contamination by blood or fluids may require customary payments to those who assist during birth (unless they are female relatives) causing some women who cannot afford these payments giving birth alone. Customary beliefs about the reasons for a difficult or complicated labour (such as social transgression or disputes) can also deter seeking health care during birth.

Sociocultural norms and customary beliefs also affect the involvement of men in pregnancy and childbirth. In many settings, taboos prevent sensitive issues concerning birth being discussed in front of men with such matters considered 'women's business' (Reed et al. 2017). For women, these taboos can prevent them accessing maternal health care for fear of being seen by male providers or male staff, particularly where there is a lack of privacy in health facilities. For men, such beliefs pose a significant barrier to participating in antenatal care or attending the birth of their children. While men, women and health providers may recognise the importance of engaging men to support the health of women and children and improve the uptake of services, few men report attending maternal health services with their partners. Taboos and gender norms contribute to the shyness, embarrassment or stigma experienced by men, together with rudeness or discouragement by health providers. The lack of a welcoming environment for men also contributes to low engagement, particularly where health facilities lack privacy (Davis et al. 2018).

## Sexually transmitted infections and cervical cancer

Across the Pacific, sexually transmitted and genital infections, including *Chlamydia Trichomonas*, *Neisseria Gonorrhoeae*, *Trichomonas Vaginalis* and syphilis, cause an unacceptable burden of disease. High rates of these infections are reported among young people and pregnant women (World Health Organization 2012). Together with HIV, high rates are also reported among women and girls who engage in transactional sex, men who have sex with men, and transgender women (Veronese et al. 2015; Kelly-Hanku et al. 2020; Hakim et al. 2021). Frequently without symptoms, many of these infections remain undiagnosed and untreated with the potential risk of onward transmission and subsequent association with adverse pregnancy and birth outcomes (including infertility, ectopic pregnancy, infertility, preterm birth, low birth weight and perinatal mortality). Published studies describing the sociocultural implications of infertility or subfertility in the Pacific are limited (Reekie et al. 2019), However, they are likely to be significant, particularly for women whose status and roles are closely linked to motherhood (see Fehoko and Shaw, Chapter 8. See Box 6.1).

The sociocultural drivers of sexually transmitted infection in the Pacific are similar to those already described above. Despite awareness of the importance of condoms to prevent transmission, use is low in many settings due to: cultural taboos that limit discussion about sexual health; the limited agency of girls and women to negotiate condom use with partners; the belief that condoms reduce sexual pleasure or interrupt sex; attitudes that condoms imply promiscuity or lack of trust in a partner; shame and stigma associated with pre- or extra-marital sex; and the judgemental attitudes of health providers and other staff where condoms are accessed (Mitchell and Bell 2020).

**Box 6.1 A reflection from Papua New Guinea: Dr Pinip Wapi:**

I see so much infertility in the community. Lots of women come to see me in clinic about getting pregnant. Often they have been married for many years and haven't been able to fall pregnant. We often find that women have had recurrent infections without any symptoms. In Papua New Guinea, we have a bride price system where the groom's family 'exchanges' cash or goods in return for marriage. This system places a lot of pressure on women to get pregnant. If they are unable to get pregnant, this can result in stigma, discrimination and an increased risk of domestic violence. Husbands might say, 'I paid your bride price, why are you not getting pregnant?' If there is a sexually transmitted infection causing infertility, this may have come from the husband due to previous relationships or extra marital affairs. However, the men think it's the women's fault. Women are always blamed for any infertility.

In many Pacific countries the control of sexually transmitted infections, such as *Chlamydia Trichomonas* and *Neiesseria Gonorrhoeae*, has relied on health promotion campaigns and individual-based case management. For example, in Fiji a national campaign has focused on promoting increased use of condoms and improving early detection and treatment of sexually transmitted infections (Fiji Ministry of Health 2016). In Vanuatu, a community theatre company has stimulated an increase in demand for sexual and reproductive health services, by highlighting and tackling these issues through theatre (Wan Smolbag Theatre Company 2021). With limited access to accurate laboratory testing, the management of sexually transmitted infections in many Pacific countries continues to be based on the now outdated World Health Organization recommendation for syndromic management, with little impact on infection rates (Vallely et al. 2017). In the absence of effective prevention and management strategies at community level, new approaches to the clinical management of sexually transmitted infections are being explored within the region. However, many of these adopt a clinical focus, reaching only those who access health services.

The Pacific has among the highest burden of cervical cancer globally. Cervical cancer is a disease of inequity; more than 85% of the global burden of cervical cancer occurs in low- and middle-income countries, where human papillomavirus vaccination, cervical screening and effective treatment for pre-cancer and cancer are largely unavailable (Bray et al. 2018). In the absence of cancer registers, mortality rates are based on estimates, with the highest estimated rate being in Papua New Guinea, where mortality is at least ten times higher than its closest neighbour, Australia (Bray et al. 2018). Limited health service infrastructure for screening and management of cervical cancer is an important contributor to morbidity and mortality, however even where cervical screening is available (usually Pap smears that require a clinical examination and sophisticated laboratory cytology) there are several barriers to women accessing services or seeking care early. Taboos regarding discussion of sex contribute to low awareness or missed opportunities to talk about cervical cancer and screening in clinical settings. The association of cervical cancer with sexually transmitted infection also contributes to shame and stigma, inhibiting care-seeking (McPherson et al. 2019). Cultural beliefs that the reproductive tract is sacred and only to be shared with husbands has also been described as a barrier to screening, in addition to fear of the procedure itself and/or of a cancer diagnosis. The introduction of new technologies such as HPV screening with the use of a self-collected samples, is offering a significant way forward to address both the shame and stigma of a clinical examination as well as the burdensome health system requirements of other, now redundant, approaches to screening in the region (Camara et al. 2021; Nguyen et al. 2022).

Within this context, human papillomavirus vaccination promises a way forward to protect against cervical cancer. However, complex social and cultural factors play a part in understanding the experience and interpretation of cervical cancer (Kelly-Hanku et al. 2018). Recent work in Papua New Guinea has demonstrated a limited understanding of cervical cancer and its cause (Kelly-Hanku et al. 2018), although high acceptability of human papillomavirus vaccination exists (Kelly-Hanku et al. 2019a). Cultural norms and taboos have important implications for vaccination campaigns and related health promotion programs. In Papua New Guinea, young people (an important population to be reached with vaccination) expressed a need for information about human papillomavirus as a sexually transmitted infection as part of efforts to prevent cancer; in contrast, however, parents and older community members (the target population to provide consent for their children), felt messaging should focus only on the prevention of cervical cancer rather than on more sensitive issues (Kelly-Hanku et al. 2019b). Outside of this setting there has been little research to understand girls' and women's knowledge, acceptability or experiences with human papillomavirus vaccination. Despite this, national vaccination programmes are underway in several Pacific countries, with Fiji and the Cook Islands leading the way with high population coverage (Ekeroma et al. 2019).

## Conclusion

Multiple factors contribute to poor sexual and reproductive health outcomes experienced by communities in the Pacific Islands region. Initiatives implemented to address these issues are often limited to individual-level behaviour-change projects, and there is need for greater community and youth-led responses to drive local initiatives embedded within relevant cultural contexts (Bell et al. 2018). Grass roots initiatives across the Pacific have been shown to be effective in improving sexual and reproductive health and well-being of the community and are essential to sustaining and expanding these efforts. Further research driven and led by Pacific scholars, clinicians, experts and community members is needed to better understand the needs, preferences and barriers that contribute to poor sexual and reproductive health outcomes, and generate data that can be used to measure change and progress.

## References

Bell, S., et al., 2018. Youth-centred research to help prevent and mitigate the adverse health and social impacts of pregnancy amongst young Papua New Guineans. *Reproductive Health Matters*, 26, 5–12. doi:10.1080/09688080.2018.1512297

Bray, F., et al., 2018. Global cancer statistics 2018: GLOBOCAN estimates of incidence and mortality worldwide for 36 cancers in 185 countries. *CA: a cancer journal for clinicians*, 68, 394–424. doi:10.3322/caac.21492

Buchanan-Aruwafu, H., 2007. Youth vulnerability to HIV in the Pacific. *Cultures and contexts matter: understanding and preventing HIV in the Pacific*, 71, 128.

Camara, H., et al., 2021. Self-collection for HPV-based cervical screening: A qualitative evidence meta-synthesis. *BMC Public Health*, 21, 1503. doi:10.1186/s12889-021-11554-6

Cammock, R., et al., 2018. Awareness and use of family planning methods among iTaukei women in Fiji and New Zealand. *Australia and New Zealand Journal of Public Health*, 42, 365–371. doi:10.1111/1753-6405.12761

Davis, J., et al., 2018. Expectant fathers' participation in antenatal care services in Papua New Guinea: A qualitative inquiry. *BMC Pregnancy and Childbirth*, 18, 138. doi:10.11 86/s12884-018-1759-4

Dawson, A., et al., 2021. How do Pacific Island countries add up on contraception, abortion and reproductive coercion? Guidance from the Guttmacher report on investing in sexual and reproductive health. *Reproductive Health*, 18, 68. doi:10.1186/s12 978-021-01122-x

Ekeroma, A., et al., 2019. Cancer management in the Pacific region: A report on innovation and good practice. *The Lancet Oncology*, 20, e493–e502. doi:10.1016/S14 70-2045(19)30414-0

Fiji Ministry of Health, 2016. *Republic of Fiji national strategic action plan on HIV and STIs 2016-2020*. Suva: Fiji Ministry of Health.

Fiji Women's Crisis Centre, 2013. *Somebody's life, everybody's business! National research on women's health and life experiences in Fiji (2010/2011): A survey exploring the prevalence, incidence and attitudes to intimate partner violence in Fiji*. Suva: Fiji Women's Crisis Centre.

Gilbert, K., et al., 2016. *Addressing preventable maternal mortality and morbidity: The determinants and consequences of unsafe abortion in Solomon Islands*. Melbourne: Ministry of Health and Medical Services Solomon Islands, Solomon Islands Planned Parenthood Association, Monash University, Burnet Institute.

Gupta, S., et al., 2020. Community attitudes and gendered influences on decision making around contraceptive implant use in rural Papua New Guinea. *Reproductive Health*, 17, 136. doi:10.1186/s12978-020-00985-w

Hakim, A.J., et al., 2021. High prevalence of chlamydia and gonorrhea and the need for sexually transmitted infection testing among men who have sex with men and transgender women in Papua New Guinea. *Sexually Transmitted Diseases*, 48 (2), 109–117. doi:10.1097/OLQ.0000000000001300

Imtishal, M. and Mohammadnezhad, M., 2021. Male partners and medical staff's perception on contributing factors of family planning (FP) in Fiji. *Heliyon*, 7, e06068. doi:10.1016/j.heliyon.2021.e06068

Institute for Health Metrics and Evaluation, 2017. *Global burden of disease study*. Seattle: Institute for Health Metrics and Evaluation.

Kelly, A., et al., 2010. Gendered talk about sex, sexual relationships and HIV among young people in Papua New Guinea. *Culture, Health & Sexuality*, 12, 221–232. doi: 10.1080/13691050903181107

Kelly-Hanku, A., et al., 2018. Ambiguous bodies, uncertain diseases: knowledge of cervical cancer in Papua New Guinea. *Ethnicity & Health*, 23 (6), 659–681. doi:10.1080/13557858.2017.1283393

Kelly-Hanku, A., et al., 2019a. HPV vaccination in Papua New Guinea to prevent cervical cancer in women: Gender, sexual morality, outsiders and the de-feminization of the HPV vaccine. *Papillomavirus Research*, 8, 100171. doi:10.1016/j.pvr.2019.100171

Kelly-Hanku, A., et al., 2019b. Health communication messaging about HPV vaccine in Papua New Guinea. *Health Education Journal*, 78, 946–957. doi:10.1177%2F0017896919856657

Kelly-Hanku, A., et al., 2020. Factors associated with HIV and syphilis infection among female sex workers in three cities in Papua New Guinea. *Sexual Health*. 17 (4), 311–320. doi:10.1071/SH19218

Kennedy, E., et al., 2013a. Addressing early and unintended *pregnancy in the Pacific: the information and service delivery needs of adolescents in Vanuatu. Policy brief*. Melbourne: Burnet Institute, Women's and Children's Health Knowledge Hub.

Kennedy, E.C., et al., 2013b. 'Be kind to young people so they feel at home': A qualitative study of adolescents' and service providers' perceptions of youth-friendly sexual and reproductive health services in Vanuatu. *BMC Health Services Research*, 13, 455. doi:10.1186/1472-6963-13-455

Kennedy, E.C., et al., 2014. 'These issues aren't talked about at home': A qualitative study of the sexual and reproductive health information preferences of adolescents in Vanuatu. *BMC Public Health*, 14, 770. doi:10.1186/1471-2458-14-770

McMillan, K. and Worth, H., 2011. The impact of socio-cultural context on young people's condom use: Evidence from two Pacific Island countries. *Culture, Health & Sexuality*, 13, 313–326. doi:10.1080/13691058.2010.529945

McPherson, G.S., Fairbairn-Dunlop, P., and Payne, D., 2019. Overcoming barriers to cervical screening among Pacific women: A narrative review. *Health Equity*, 3, 22–29. doi:10.1089/heq.2018.0076

Mitchell, E. and Bell, S., 2020. Premarital relationships and condom use among young people in Suva, Fiji. *Sexual Health*, 17, 337–343. doi:10.1071/SH20040

Mitchell, E. and Bennett, L.R., 2020. Pressure and persuasion: Young Fijian women's experiences of sexual and reproductive coercion in romantic relationships. *Violence Against Women*, 26, 1555–1573. doi:10.1177/1077801219882505

National Department of Health, 2019. *Provincial and district health profiles*. Port Moresby: PNG National Department of Health.

Nguyen, D.T.N., et al., 2022. Towards the elimination of cervical cancer in low-income and lower-middle-income countries: Modelled evaluation of the effectiveness and cost-effectiveness of point-of-care HPV self-collected screening and treatment in Papua New Guinea. *BMJ Global Health*, 7 (3), e007380. doi:10.1136/bmjgh-2021-007380

Peach, E., et al., 2021. Risk factors and knowledge associated with high unintended pregnancy rates and low family planning use among pregnant women in Papua New Guinea. *Scientific Reports*, 11, 1222. doi:10.1038/s41598-020-79103-6

Pio, F.H. and Nosa, V., 2020. Health literacy of Samoan mothers and their experiences with health professionals. *Journal of Primary Health Care*, 12, 57–63. doi:10.1071/HC19026

Reed, S.J., et al., 2017. Honoring motherhood: The meaning of childbirth for Tongan women. *MCN, The American Journal of Maternal/Child Nursing*, 42 (3), 146–152. doi:10.1097/NMC.0000000000000328

Reekie, J., et al., 2019. Risk of ectopic pregnancy and tubal infertility following gonorrhea and chlamydia infections. *Clinical Infectious Diseases*, 69, 1621–1623. doi:10.1093/cid/ciz145

Robbers, G., et al., 2019. Maternal and newborn health indicators in Papua New Guinea–2008–2018. *Sexual and Reproductive Health Matters*, 27, 52–68. doi:10.1080/26410397.2019.1686199

Sully, E.A., et al., 2019. *Adding it up: Investing in sexual and reproductive health 2019*. New York: Guttmacher Institute

UNFPA, 2021. *My body is my body, my life is my life. Sexual and reproductive health and rights of young people in Asia and the Pacific*. Bangkok: UNFPA Asia Pacific Regional Office.

Vallely, L.M., Homiehombo, P., Kelly-Hanku, A., Vallely, A., et al., 2015. Childbirth in a rural highlands community in Papua New Guinea: A descriptive study. *Midwifery*, 31, 380–387. doi:10.1016/j.midw.2014.11.002

Vallely, L.M., Homiehombo, P., Kelly-Hanku, A., and Whittaker, A., 2015. Unsafe abortion requiring hospital admission in the Eastern Highlands of Papua New Guinea: A descriptive study of women's and health care workers' experiences. *Reproductive Health*, 12, 22. doi:10.1186/s12978-015-0015-x

Vallely, L.M., et al., 2017. Performance of syndromic management for the detection and treatment of genital *Chlamydia trachomatis*, *Neisseria gonorrhoeae* and *Trichomonas vaginalis* among women attending antenatal, well woman and sexual health clinics in Papua New Guinea: A cross-sectional study. *BMJ Open*, 7, e018630. doi:10.1136/bmjopen-2017-018630

Veronese, V., et al., 2015. Sexually transmitted infections among transgender people and men who have sex with men in Port Vila, Vanuatu. *Western Pacific Surveillance and Response Journal*, 6, 55–59. doi:10.5365/wpsar.2014.5.1.003

Wan Smolbag Theatre Company, 2021. *Wan Smolbag* [online]. Vanuatu. Available from: https://www.wansmolbag.org/film/ [Accessed 19 January 2022].

White, A.L., Mann, E.S., and Larkan, F., 2018. 'You just have to learn to keep moving on': Young women's experiences with unplanned pregnancy in the Cook Islands. *Culture, Health & Sexuality*, 20 (7), 731–745. doi:10.1080/13691058.2017.1371336

Wilson, A., et al., 2020. Improving the quality of maternal and newborn care in the Pacific region: A scoping review. *The Lancet Regional Health-Western Pacific*, 3, 100028. doi:10.1016/j.lanwpc.2020.100028

Winn-Dix, E.A., Nathan, S.A., and Rawstorne, P., 2016. Informing the introduction of contraceptive implants in the Pacific: A mixed methods study of contraceptive beliefs and behaviours in Tonga. *Australia and New Zealand Journal of Public Health*, 40 (2), 115–119. doi:10.1111/1753-6405.12494

World Health Organization, 2012. *Global incidence and prevalence of selected curable sexually transmitted infections* [online]. Geneva: World Health Organization. Available from: http://www.who.int/reproductivehealth/publications/rtis/stiestimates/en/ [Accessed 19 January 2022].

# 7 Grassroots action for improved menstrual health and educational justice with girls in East Kwaio, Solomon Islands

*Dorothy Esau, Michelle Redman-MacLaren, Stephanie Wheeler, Relmah Baritama Harrington and Karen Cheer*

*E'uta nauku etania taunga'inga lo'ori. Latagu ni Dorothy Esau, nauku lane fana mule farisi Na 2001, nauku nanai fe'enia ta'aagu I fataia fana akwale farisi, sui ma nauku sakaa no fani asi ma ku nanai ai fana fiu farisi, nauku leka kwairiu mola fani asi ma fataia. Usugani furifuri nauku leka fana taugaingai 'ii Atoifi Hospital, nauku leka maku daria te welegeni lari'i lo siria tala, ngai'e orimai fa'asia lanenga ana na usugani mola. Nauku aga fana ma ku orisia? 'E fe'ua io orimai fa'asia lanenga amu, suria ame nigi uwa na alata fana lanenga ani sui. Ngai e dua nau na kwaimandaenga, 'e iria ngai e toobi, sui ma mele ka alafu la'a mola. Ngai'e alafu suria nga labena, ma lefu ngai 'e lane ai ... 'Ola etaeta ngai iria, ngai ame to'ona bata fana sugalana suingi, fana ani ru'ufia, suria nga kabilato ana ta esia, ma ngai ne agea, ngai ka leka no fa'asia lanega ana, sui ma ngai ame to'ona kabilato le'a fana ngai ani ru'ufia, ngai na alata ngai e tobi ma abu e lago na rufi ana, ma alata ru'uru'uwa gila agasia nga abu na rufi ana ma gila ka osa'ania, ma ngai ne mau maka ori no'o fani efii fa'asia lanengaana. Sui ma ngai e iria lefu fana ani wasia labena e amoe, lefu fana ani dua nga kabilato ana ka amoe la'a mola. Ma ngai ne noniri'a fana leka no'o fana lane nga. Alata nauku longoa nga sisifonga lo fa'asia welageni lo'o, nauku manata fa'aburu, suria nau la'a mola ku leka ubulai sui no'o. Ma ngai na ku manta fana taunga'i nga lo na Menstrual hygiene program lo fana aku kwaiboni na ru'uru'u geni na lanenga 'I east kwaio ani gila leka fana lanenga, sui ma ngai mala ola fana nanau lai fana east kwaio school, sui ma ngai te kwaiboni la'a mola fana ani gila usim kabilota fooru. Nga sisifonga lo'ori agu siria taungai agu fe'enia ta'aagu I kwaio. Fana ani agea nga lamaduanga fana ru'uaagu ma fuigeni agu I kwaio fana to'orule'a nga.*

*Dorothy Esau*

Every morning I used to walk to work; I move up and down between the mountains and the coast living in both these worlds. One day, I met a young girl coming back from school early at 10am. I asked, 'Why are you coming back from school, it's not the right time.' She answered me sadly, 'I'm menstruating.' She told me she hasn't got money to buy underwear to protect her and without them her pads would fall off, so she had to go home and miss school. And she hasn't got any proper pads to use, that's why blood stained her skirt. When other students saw the stain, they laughed at her, she was afraid and embarrassed and

DOI: 10.4324/9781003142072-9

> left. Worse, at school they haven't got any bathroom to help her change her pads and wash her body for her privacy. She doesn't want to be at school when she menstruates.
>
> Dorothy Esau

This account, shared in Kwaio and translated into English, is the story of how one determined and committed woman from East Kwaio, Solomon Islands, used a chance encounter with a young girl to be the impetus for her, and our, work with local community members to achieve improved menstrual health for this young schoolgirl, and all women and girls. But it is more than that. It is a story of bringing about local transformation to ensure both reproductive and educational justice for girls.[1]

## Menstruation in East Kwaio

East Kwaio is located on the east coast of the island province of Malaita, Solomon Islands and is home to approximately 10,000 people who live almost entirely in villages supported by a subsistence economy. East Kwaio is mountainous, with steep slopes rising from a coastal fringe of beaches and coral reefs. Twice weekly, a light aircraft services the grass airstrip at Atoifi Adventist Hospital and a ship, carrying passengers and goods, services villages fortnightly. There are no roads. People paddle dugout canoes or walk between villages and speak Kwaio, one of over 70 Solomon Islands' languages.

Religion and spirituality determine daily life here, as in much of the country, and in the Pacific more generally. Every village on the coastal fringe belongs to a Christian denomination brought to the Solomon Islands during colonisation; independence was gained from Great Britain in 1978. Everyone who lives in a coastal village is either a member of, or follows the rules of, the Christian denomination to which the village belongs. In the mountains of East Kwaio, most people have chosen not to adopt Christianity, instead retaining traditional ancestral beliefs and practices. People live on their own tribal land in small family-sized hamlets, cleared from dense rainforest and connected to gardens and other hamlets by a network of walking trails.

The physical layout of a Kwaio mountain hamlet is determined by the biological, socio-cultural and spiritual process of menstruation. Each hamlet has three main dwellings: a *bisi* (menstrual house, see Figure 7.1); an *ifi* (family house); and a *tau* (men's house), situated a few metres apart, all three within full sight of one another. A line of low shrubs designates the physical and cosmological boundary between the female-family-male sections of the hamlet. When a woman/girl menstruates, she is regarded as *abu* (sacred) and stays in the bisi. When a man makes a sacrifice to the ancestral spirits, for example the sacrifice of a *fo'ota* (sacred pig), he is also regarded as abu and stays in the tau. When a woman/girl completes her monthly menstrual cycle and/or when a man completes his time in the tau, they return to a non-sacred state known as *mola*. All

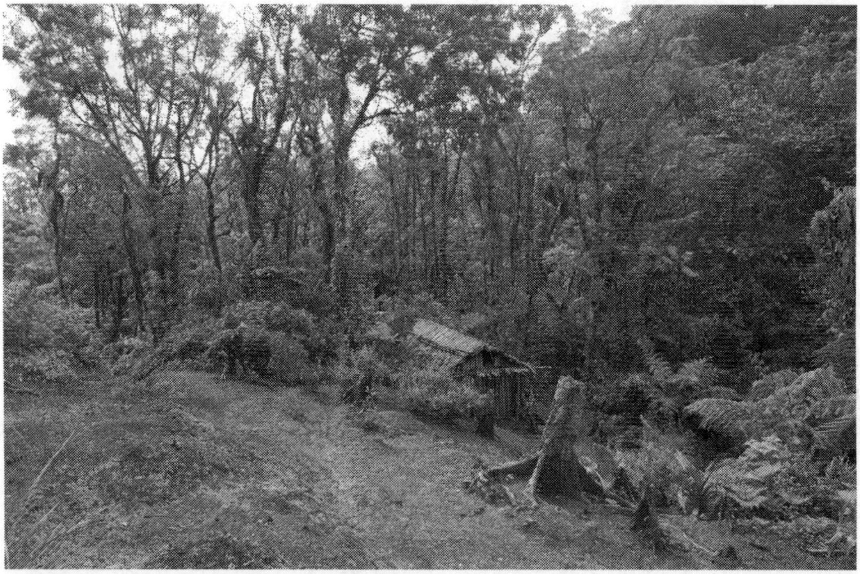

*Figure 7.1* Bisi (menstrual house) in East Kwaio.

Source: Photo by Tommy Esau. Used with permission.

people in mola stay in the ifi. There are no restrictions on knowing which people are abu at any time, indeed this information is essential to know where people will be and to plan kin and tribal activities that meet collective responsibilities to both the living and the ancestors. Menstruation is openly discussed between kin and women/girls stay in either the bisi or ifi (depending on where they are in their menstrual cycle) to safely manage these responsibilities. Menstrual blood is not tolerated in communal areas since this would make the ancestors angry and could cause harm or even death to a family member (Akin 2003). Women/girls manage these *abunga* (taboos) by staying in the bisi when they are menstruating. Communal female toilets and communal female water sources are connected to the larger category of female bodily waste, adjacent to the bisi. Abunga are managed collectively, with no shame or stigma associated with menstruation in Kwaio hamlets.

In contrast to the mountain hamlets, menstruation does not determine the physical layout of a Kwaio Christian village. Each Christian Kwaio village has a single church building surrounded by family dwellings. The people who live in these dwellings can be from different tribal groups, yet everyone speaks the same Kwaio language. There is no bisi; women/girls are not regarded as sacred when they menstruate and as such there are no designated cosmological boundaries. Menstruation is not openly discussed, and individual women/girls are expected to manage menstruation alone. In these villages there are communal female toilets/toilet areas, often a long way from women's houses. There are no specific water sources for women/girls to use during menstruation and/or for menstrual health and hygiene. Kwaio girls in these settings are often unprepared for menstruation, lacking accurate and timely knowledge, safe and affordable materials, and/or access to adequate and private water and sanitation facilities.

## Kwaio girls are not alone

In the Pacific, and in East Kwaio, the biological realities of menarche, the first menstruation, and subsequent cyclic ovarian function that persists until menopause to signal the end of a woman's reproductive life, are often embedded within and interpreted through a cultural or spiritual lens (Akin 2003; Mohamed et al. 2018; Maulingin-Gumbaketi et al. 2021); cultural explanations of menstruation, ways of thinking about the body and its cyclical bleeding still dominate many traditional contexts (Dammery 2016). Tales about menstruation abound, often characterising menstrual blood as sacred, a gift from the gods, or a punishment for sin, but always as magical and powerful (Tan et al. 2017).

Despite the universal nature of the biological process of menses, girls across the Pacific, and elsewhere, continue to be ill-prepared for menarche and subsequent management of menstruation (Redman-MacLaren et al. 2018; UNICEF 2019). The lack of basic knowledge about puberty and menstruation among girls, especially in low- and middle-income countries may contribute to early and unwanted pregnancy and stress and shame associated with menstruation, and make girls susceptible to reproductive tract infections from use of unhygienic sanitation products (Kiribati Ministry of Education 2018; UNICEF 2019). In the absence of good reproductive health knowledge, materials to manage menstruation, or access to adequate water, sanitation and hygiene facilities, girls face the challenge of managing their menstrual bleeding alone, with significant cultural and educational impacts, missing days from school.

## Water, sanitation and hygiene in schools in East Kwaio

Like other girls, Kwaio girls need daily access to water, sanitation and hygiene facilities to successfully manage menstrual health and hygiene and fulfil their right to education by consistently being able to attend school, irrespective of where they are in the menstrual cycle. When schoolgirls are menstruating they regularly miss school, as Dorothy's story shows. Water, sanitation and hygiene facilities are rarely found in East Kwaio. There are no church or government schools in the Kwaio Mountains. In coastal areas of East Kwaio, schools are managed by the church or the government. For the few schools with a toilet and running water, systems are rarely maintained. A small achievement was realised in one East Kwaio school where in 2019 a single tap was installed for drinking water and handwashing. Although they have been agreed to by the community, the toilets are yet to be built. In schools throughout Solomon Islands, more than 60% have no sanitation options (UNICEF and WHO 2020). Unaddressed, these gendered water, sanitation and hygiene challenges only widen the gender gap in formal education.

There are successful programmes by non-governmental agencies in some Solomon Island schools to improve access to water and sanitation, and attitudes towards menstrual health and hygiene (Abel 2020). A recent review of literature reporting water, sanitation and hygiene systems in Pacific schools identified the need to incorporate local ways of knowing and learning to ensure new systems meet the needs of girls in schools (Redman-MacLaren et al. 2018). Local level action, led by community leaders, marks an important shift towards the centralising of local wisdom and accountability often absent in Western programmes. By leading local level action for improved menstrual health challenges, we can generate sustained, positive change for girls locally. This is the approach the lead author – Dorothy – whose story starts this chapter, has undertaken with her female relatives, and which was actively supported by the other authors and collaborators.

## Kwaio women leading change

In 2019, as a group of female advocates for women and girls, we started discussing ways we might leverage our skills to respond to the obvious need for improved menstrual health and hygiene options in our East Kwaio communities. Together, Dorothy and Michelle met with members of the Baru Conservation Alliance and other community members in East Kwaio to discuss possible action and resource implications of any initiative to respond to the needs of our girls. Together with the communities and organisations, it was decided that a holistic approach was needed to promote improved menstrual hygiene, menstrual health and advocate for water, sanitation and hygiene facilities in two local schools. It was also decided that this work needed an integrated evaluation to improve future activities. Dorothy and her cousin sisters initially met with 'matrons'— married female teachers — at two schools to gauge their interest and then secure a commitment to partnering in this work. The two school principals were then invited to provide their support.[2]

## The girls at the heart of our work

The girls who participated in the project were primary and secondary school students aged 12–17 years. Key components of the project were the development and distribution of locally-made, reusable pads and delivery of education sessions about reproductive health and menstrual health and hygiene. We interviewed girls about their experiences of menstruation in East Kwaio, held feedback sessions with students, teachers and community members (including parents), and had separate evaluative discussions with girls about their experience of using the pads.

### *Component one: development and distribution of locally-made pads*

The programme started by viewing examples of handmade, reusable sanitary pads used in projects led by women leaders around the world, including from Fiji (Earth Sisters Fiji 2021). We found pad design and materials differed according to climate, facilities and dress codes and knew consideration of the East Kwaio context was important. The pads had to be soft and comfortable so girls would want to wear them and would need to provide effective protection to give girls confidence to attend school without worrying about leakage. The pads also had to be able to be hand-washed and dry efficiently in East Kwaio's humid and rainy weather, weighing the additional protection that multi-layered pads offer against drying time. We also considered the cost of providing enough pads to each girl to ensure coverage while used pads dried. We learned about polyurethane laminate, a waterproof material that can be sewn between layers of cotton to provide protection to reduce bulkiness and drying time. Polyurethane laminate material was sourced in Australia and sent to Solomon Islands.

During the early design phase of pad-making, we spoke with a woman leader and entrepreneur, Mary Elizabeth Ramosaea, Business Director of *Kaleko Steifree*. Mary leads a small enterprise making reusable menstrual pads for girls in Solomon Islands. She generously shared with us her experience of establishing *Kaleko Steifree*, invited us to visit her business and provided valuable advice on production and distribution including the importance of polyurethane laminate, the different sizes of pads required and the different levels of protection required for different days of menstruation.

Dorothy, along with Jenta and Stephanie (Dorothy's family members), began to sew the pads by hand and on an electric sewing machine purchased for the project (see Figure 7.2). Along with Dorothy, the women created and trialled

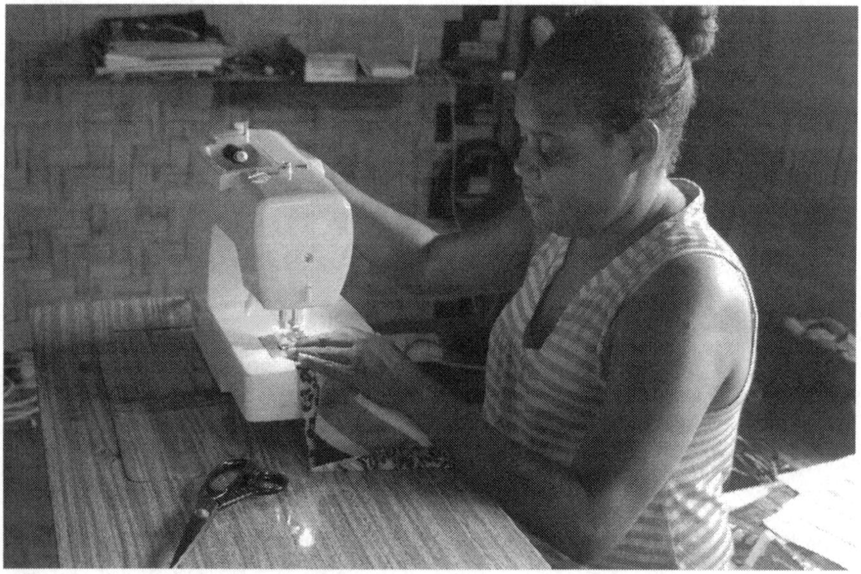

*Figure 7.2* Sewing of reusable pads in East Kwaio.

Source: Photo by Tommy Esau. Used with permission.

different designs and sizes of pads. The women shared their preferences about each design, and combined feedback into a final design. Together they established an efficient process to produce 100 pads weekly.

Across two schools, 125 girl students received a small cotton drawstring bag containing five locally-made pads and a pair of new underpants. Within four months over 600 pads had been distributed (see Table 7.1).

### *Component two: education programme*

To inform our education programme we reviewed relevant aspects of the Solomon Islands school curriculum, specifically the Science Year 9 Learner's Book (Solomon Islands Ministry of Education and Human Resources Development [MEHRD] 2013). The basic anatomical information was accurate but suggestions for managing menstruation were irrelevant to the girls in a coastal village setting. Under the heading 'Menstruation,' girls were instructed to 'make sure you have sanitary pads, napkins or tampons ready. You need to change your pad at least three times a day during menstruation' and reminded, 'Do not flush pads in toilets' (MEHRD 2013, pp. 30–31). This would be sage advice if there were sanitary pads available, there was a toilet and there was a flush option! With almost 80% of the population living in village settings with conditions such as those in East Kwaio, the inadequacy of the uncritical importation of formal knowledge systems and education curriculum from elsewhere was highlighted.

The role of teachers is critical to successful delivery of sexual and reproductive health information. It was informally reported that teachers lack confidence in teaching basic sexual and reproductive health and were concerned about cultural and religious implications, especially when a male teacher was expected to teach reproductive health to female students. Similar findings from Fiji (Ram and Mohammadenzhad 2019) and Papua New Guinea (Kokinai 2014), highlight the need to support student teachers to competently deliver the sexual and reproductive health curriculum, and for school leadership and local authorities to support teachers and promote open and accurate communication with communities.

We used this information to provide education sessions about reproductive health and menstrual health and hygiene for girls in the two schools. We invited a female doctor and female nurse from Atoifi Adventist Hospital to present in these sessions. Complementing Dorothy's expertise in engaging with women in communities, the involvement of healthcare workers added credibility to our programme, ensured girls' questions were competently answered and built rapport and relationships with female health care workers to whom the girls could reach out to in the future.

At School One, a 90-minute session was held for student girls and female teachers. The male school principal opened the programme to show his support for our work. The boys heard about the programme but although they really wanted to listen to the health workers, the girls did not want the boys to listen to their stories — they told members of our team it was a "girls" story.' Our team doctor and nurse then gave a presentation on the female reproductive system and the process of menstruation. The four girl students, female teaching staff and our programme team sat together in a circle to share, listen and ask questions. Hesitancy noted during the discussion related to the use of polyurethane laminate material, which hitherto had not been used for menstrual hygiene management in East Kwaio. Dorothy affirmed other women in Solomon Islands used this material and the team doctor confirmed polyurethane laminate was safe for use.

At School Two, the team nurse presented for 90 minutes on menstruation and reproductive health, about the importance of washing with soap and clean water as well as keeping pads clean. The challenges of cleaning and drying the pads in the village context and during rainy weather were discussed. Girls at this school (n = 28) reported enjoying the presentation. They appeared shy and only asked questions in smaller groups after the session. Girls also quizzed the project team – most of whom were long-standing village members – indicating the likelihood that girls felt uncomfortable talking in a large group, and demonstrating the value of trust built through ongoing relationships.

## What the girls told us

To develop a a more in-depth understanding of girls' experiences of menstruation in East Kwaio we held in-depth interviews with two primary school girls and two group interviews comprising of 4 and 28 girl students respectively (Table 7.1).

The in-depth and group interviews, conducted in Kwaio and Solomon Islands Pijin, followed a predetermined interview guide based upon: 1. locally identified needs; 2. a UNICEF tool (Caruso 2013); and 3. experience of conducting research in East Kwaio with women and girls across a range of health issues. Following assurances of confidentiality, rapport building discussion took place about a typical school day and favourite activities. Topics included health

*Table 7.1* Girls interviewed, pads distributed and education sessions

| *Location* | *Girls interviewed* | | *Girls who received pads* | *Number pads distributed* | *Education/feedback sessions* |
|---|---|---|---|---|---|
| School 1 | Primary | 1 | 31 | 155 | 2 |
| | Secondary | 3 | 7 | 35 | |
| School 2 | Primary | 21* | 63 | 315 | 2 |
| | Secondary | 9 | 24 | 120 | |
| **TOTAL** | | **34** | **125** | **625** | **4** |

Notes
* At School 2, 28 in a group interview comprising Primary (n = 19) and Secondary students (n = 9); Additional 2 individual interviews were with Primary students.

education; differences for boys and girls who attended school; attitudes towards menstruation; and how girls managed menstruation (Caruso 2013).

Dorothy analysed interview recordings using a close-listening method, consistent with oral communication of stories in Kwaio cultural context and audio-privileged qualitative data analysis methods (Tessier 2012).

### What girls called menstruation

The traditional term for menstruation in Kwaio is *tobinga* and is used by members of the older generation in the mountains, but not young girls in Christian villages. In the nearby hospital, nurses use the Pijin word *flaoa* (literally, flower), which is also understood by people in Kwaio to mean menstruation. Girls involved in this project, however, called menstruation both 'menses' and 'periods.' The menstrual health and hygiene sessions before the interview may have influenced use of these two English terms. While girls knew the onset of their menstruation was connected to the new moon they saw each month, they did not use a term related to the moon, as in other Solomon Islands provinces, for example Choiseul, where menstruation is referred to as girls and women 'seeing the moon.' In other Melanesian contexts, for example Papua New Guinea, the term for menstruation – *sik mun* – similarly makes reference to the illness/condition that is seen as occuring once a moon cycle or month.

### How girls experienced and managed menstruation

Girls reported menstruation bringing about mixed feelings. Some felt stressed and ashamed, especially if they were without prior knowledge. Some older girls believed younger girls should not yet have menses – girls can be laughed at if they have early menses. Other girls felt happy, thinking 'bad blood' was being removed from their body, '*samfala hapi bikos rabis blad hem aot*' and wanted to show off to the boys. When girls understood about the purpose of menstruation, and that it was normal, they welcomed its onset.

Most girls were absent from school when menstruating. They feared blood stains on their uniforms and odour that could occur: '*Samfala frait nogud blad pas lo skirt blo oketa en hem smel.*' Both fears and the risk of being laughed at keeps girls at home. Without money to buy pads, girls reported using old cloths or towels, old or new nappies, or toilet paper; some used 'double undies,' wearing two pairs of underpants. Other girls who did not even have the resources for underpants feared whatever they used, pads might fall off in public: '*Samfala frait, nogud kabilato foldaon bikos oketa no werem pant.*' Girls self-managed this fear by staying away from school. Some girls attended school because they could wash themselves in their village and use pads at school: '*Samfala gele save go skul bikos oketa swim gud and usim pad.*' Overall, the girls preferred to manage their menses at home as schools involved in this project had no private facilities where girls could change their pads or wash.

## Girls' feedback about the pads

We initially distributed a pack of five pads to each girl, but some girls reported five pads were insufficient. Further stories with girls identified two key reasons for this. First, distributing pads to one schoolgirl in a collective society often means the girl must share pads with female relatives. Material possessions are considered collective property in this social context, with a novel product being particularly prized. While five pads may meet the biological needs of a single girl, when each girl is considered in their family context, five was insufficient for the collective need. To better meet the need of individual girls, the project needed to broaden distribution to ensure equitable access to period products for all menstruating women and girls.

Second, girls had trouble drying pads in time for their next use, especially during wet weather or if there were no private places to hang pads in the sun. Girls reported trying to dry their pads inside their houses. We learned that we needed to integrate training on laundering and care of pads. In addition to sufficient sunlight, girls needed to be able to dry their pads in an area separate from communal space, particularly away from areas where visiting *kastom* friends and family stay.

Even with the aid of pads, girls also struggled to manage their menstruation at school; there was nowhere to change or wash the pads. What to do with used pads was another concern: one girl carried her used pad in an old plastic bag, but few girls have access to plastic in these village settings, nor did we wish to encourage potentially harmful environmental practices. We recognise that consistent availability of safe and culturally appropriate water, sanitation and hygiene infrastructure at schools is required to meet this need. Baru Conservation Alliance advocates for the provision of these services, cognisant of the needs of young girls and women. We plan to address a small component of this larger issue by making and distributing small polyurethane laminate-lined bags for girls to carry used pads, to ensure they can hygienically bring them home from school.

## A systems approach to menstrual hygiene in East Kwaio

Women and girls in the Pacific with access to menstrual health and hygiene services, products and facilities enjoy a higher level of health, dignity, autonomy and control over their lives (Criterion Institute and Pacific RISE 2018). They can also fulfil their right to education. Through the work we have undertaken we have learned, however, that the production of pads is only one component of a much wider solution to this issue. This project has highlighted the need to plan and implement future work with a broader systems approach that ensures menstrual health and hygiene is integrated into cultural, family and educational systems and infrastructure.

Families and communities need to be at the centre of menstrual health and hygiene initiatives introducing and normalising reusable sanitary pads. One girl from a Christian village reported that her brother brought a reusable pad from a washing line and asked her, 'What is this?' This was shameful for both the boy and girl; the shame could be avoided if there was broader communication about the pads. The role of mothers/parents is critical to increasing acceptability of menstrual health and hygiene management, reducing stigma and ensuring girls have equitable educational opportunities with boys in their families and communities. Feedback to parents, schools and community about the project was an important first step to assist in supporting the acceptability of menstrual health and hygiene management.

We had originally designed the school awareness-raising component of the project to include education for boys, as menstrual education is an integral part of normal human physiology and had been shown to be an effective strategy in reducing stigma and shame in other Pacific contexts (Mohamed et al. 2018). It also created a supportive environment within which girls could feel safe and empowered to continue their education during menstruation. Unfortunately, we were unable to expand the programme to include boys due to time and resource constraints. We were, however, able to engage with male community leaders including Kwaio village chiefs, who provided cultural insights into traditional perspectives of menstrual hygiene and encouraged the teachers to promote menstrual health and hygiene with the participating schoolgirls.

## Where to next?

Through this work and our ongoing relationships in the community, we continue to advocate with village leaders to prioritise water, sanitation and hygiene facilities for all girls in East Kwaio, especially those at school. Building on an initial, largely unremarkable conversation with a girl on her way home with a blood-stained skirt, Dorothy was able to galvanise support for this project. Now the evidence generated in the project has provided impetus for action by others. One of the two schools has purchased its own sewing machine and is making its own pads. We have extended our work and commenced work with girls and their families in a mountain hamlet with a small community-run school. In this work, we are exploring menstruation management options and trialling *kabilato*-style pads: reusable cloth pads that can be threaded on to traditional kabilato belts made of lawyer cane (*Calamus Arecaceae)* that don't need underpants. From this small project we are supporting and fostering other locally-grown and locally-led initiatives to address gender and health in contemporary Kwaio, drawing on and valuing beliefs and practices of the past.

Our story provides an example of how community-based, local level action can make a real and genuine difference in the lives of girls. Ensuring our daughters have access to menstrual health and hygiene services as part of an integrated approach to sexual and reproductive health, as we have illustrated, is essential to reduce school absenteeism or withdrawal from school, and progress efforts in gender equity. It is also a story about how partnerships, led by those closest to the issue, in this case from within the communities in the Solomon Islands, can influence change.

We have much work to still do, and hope that sharing our story encourages others to consider what they can do in their schools, and in their communities, to improve the health and educational opportunities of girls in our region, and beyond. Menstruation should never limit Pacific girls, nor result in shame or stigma or restrict their access to formal education.

## Notes

1 We acknowledge the valuable cultural advice and ongoing support provided for our menstrual health and hygiene work by Chief Esau Kekeubata, David MacLaren and Tommy Esau.

2 Funding was made available from the College of Medicine and Dentistry, James Cook University, for sewing machines and materials to produce sanitary pads and to pay for Dorothy's time to manage the programme, wages for Dorothy's cousins to sew the pads and printing and communication costs. After addressing cultural protocols, and to ensure the safety and well-being of the schoolgirls and their families while addressing this culturally sensitive health issue, ethical approval was granted by ethics committees of Atoifi Hospital and James Cook University.

## References

Abel, M., 2020. *WASH in schools implementation guidelines*. Melbourne: Live & Learn Environmental Education.

Akin, D., 2003. Concealment, confession, and innovation in Kwaio women's taboos. *American Ethnologist*, 30 (3), 381–400.

Caruso, B., 2013. *WASH in schools empowers girls' education: Tools for assessing menstrual hygiene management in schools*. New York: UNICEF.

Criterion Institute and Pacific RISE, 2018. *Unlocking the opportunity in the Pacific menstrual health market* [online]. Available from: https://mhm.pacificrise.org/wp-content/uploads/2019/03/Unlocking-the-opportunity-in-the-Pacific-menstrual-health-market19March.pdf [Accessed 29 June 2021].

Dammery, S., 2016. *First blood: A cultural study of menarche*. Melbourne: Monash University Publishing.

Earth Sisters Fiji, 2021. *Earth sisters: Beautiful reusables* [online]. Available from: https://www.earthsistersfiji.com/ [Accessed 29 June 2021].

Kiribati Ministry of Education, 2018. *Breaking down barriers: Coming of age, becoming the change*. Tarawa, Kiribati: Ministry of Education.

Kokinai, C., 2014. *Seventh-day Adventist education system response to HIV and AIDS in Papua New Guinea: A case study*. Thesis (Master of Philosophy). Pacific Adventist University, Port Moresby.

Maulingin-Gumbaketi, E., et al., 2021. 'Making of a Strong Woman': a constructivist grounded theory of the experiences of young women around menarche in Papua New Guinea. *BMC Women's Health*, 21 (1), 144. doi:10.1186/s12905-021-01229-0

MEHRD (Solomon Islands Ministry of Education and Human Resources Development), 2013. *Solomon Islands science year 9 learner's book*. Melbourne: Pearson Education.

Mohamed, Y., et al., 2018. A qualitative exploration of menstruation-related restrictive practices in Fiji, Solomon Islands and Papua New Guinea. *PLoS ONE*, 13 (12), e0208224.

Ram, S. and Mohammadenzhad, M., 2019. Sexual and reproductive health in schools in Fiji: A qualitative study of teachers' perceptions. *Health Education*, 120 (1), 55–71. doi:10.1108/HE-02-2019-0005

Redman-MacLaren, M., et al., 2018. Water, sanitation and hygiene systems in Pacific Island schools to promote the health and education of girls and children with disability: A systematic scoping review. *Journal of Water, Sanitation and Hygiene for Development*, 8 (3), 386–401. doi:10.2166/washdev.2018.274

Tan, D.A., Haththotuwa, R., and Fraser, I.S., 2017. Cultural aspects and mythologies surrounding menstruation and abnormal uterine bleeding. *Best Practice & Research Clinical Obstetrics & Gynaecology*, 40, 121–133. doi:10.1016/j.bpobgyn.2016.09.015

Tessier, S., 2012. From field notes, to transcripts, to tape recordings: Evolution or combination? *International Journal of Qualitative Methods*, 11 (4), 446–460. doi:10.1177/160940691201100410

UNICEF, 2019. *Guidance on menstrual health and hygiene* [online]. Available from: https://www.unicef.org/media/91341/file/UNICEF-Guidance-menstrual-health-hygiene-2019.pdf [Accessed 29 June 2021].

UNICEF and WHO, 2020. *Progress on drinking water, sanitation and hygiene in schools: Special focus on COVID-19* [online]. Available from https://www.who.int/docs/default-source/wash-documents/progress-of-drinking-water-sanitation-and-hygiene-in-schools---special-focus-on-covid-19.pdf?sfvrsn=d5b40ebd_6&download=true [Accessed 29 June 2021].

# 8 From burdens to blessings: A Pacific perspective on infertility and assisted reproductive technologies in Aotearoa | New Zealand

*Edmond S. Fehoko and Rhonda M. Shaw*

## Introduction

Medical infertility is commonly defined as the incapacity 'to achieve a pregnancy after 12 months or more of regular unprotected sexual intercourse' (WHO n.d.). Global estimates vary, but recent studies indicate that infertility affects 15% of the world's population of reproductive age (Sun et al. 2019). In high-income countries such as Aotearoa | New Zealand and Australia, infertility affects between one in six couples to one in five couples (Fertility Society of Australia 2016; Goodman et al. 2020). Assisted reproductive technologies can support individuals and couples to bypass and overcome a range of infertility challenges in the hope of having a biologically related family. Over the last four decades, the use of these technologies has steadily increased, with approximately 530,000 babies being born each year as a result (ESHRE 2018). Despite the increased availability of many assisted reproductive technologies internationally, disparities related to socio-economic factors and patient care continue to impact outcomes and access to fertility treatment and reproductive services (McQueen et al. 2015; Mourad et al. 2019). In this chapter, we examine some of the barriers facing Pacific Islander women in Aotearoa | NZ when accessing and utilising fertility treatment services.

## Fertility care

Pacific peoples comprise 8.1% of the Aotearoa | NZ population, and comprise many different groups (including Tongan, Fijian, Niuean, Samoan, Cook Islanders, Tuvaluan and Tokelauan), each with their own cultural values, beliefs, language, social structure, identity and history. Family is the foundation and cornerstone for all Pacific groups and communities (Meleisea and Schoeffel 1998). While birth rates were as high as 2.94 births per woman in 2001, today they have fallen to 2.19 births per woman, still higher than the birth rate of 1.75 births per woman for the general Aotearoa | NZ population (Statistics New Zealand 2019). While Pacific women have more childen, they do so at a younger age. In Aotearoa | NZ the median childbearing age for Pacific women is 27.5 years compared to 31 years for women of European descent (Statistics New Zealand 2019).

DOI: 10.4324/9781003142072-10

Moreover, while Pacific women are more likely to have children at a younger age, and are therefore less likely than women of European descent to experience age-related fertility risks, they are susceptible to several other risk factors associated with infertility.

There are many causes of infertility. For Pacific Islanders two common causes relate to reproductive tract infections and obesity. *Chlamydia trachomatis* is a sexually transmitted infection that is common among young Pacific Islanders of reproductive age in Aotearoa | NZ. Statistics show that Pacific women have the second highest rate of Chlamydia (2012 per 100,000) across all population groups in Aotearoa | NZ (Institute of Environmental Science and Research 2019). Left untreated, Chlamydia can lead to pelvic inflammatory disease and tubal factor infertility in women. Being underweight or having an obese Body Mass Index (BMI) have been identified as risk factors for infertility (Righarts et al. 2015). While 30% of the Aotearoa | NZ adult population is considered obese (BMI >30kg/m2), Pacific people in Aotearoa | NZ have an especially high prevalence of obesity and this rate increases with age, with a BMI over 35kg/m2 being two- to four-fold higher than for Aotearoa | NZ Europeans (Tremellen et al. 2017). Having a BMI over 32 kg/m2 is typically cited as the single biggest risk factor that results in poor health outcomes, reduced quality of life and increased health care costs, and is also considered a major contributor to infertility (Farquhar and Gillett 2006; Tupai-Firestone et al. 2016).

In Aotearoa | NZ there are three main providers of fertility services (Fertility Associates, Fertility Plus, Repromed). All three offer private and publicly funded treatment. Government funded fertility treatment is dependent on strict clinical criteria that restrict access to assisted reproductive technologies to women aged 39 years or younger, non-smokers, and those with a BMI within the range of 18–32 kg/m2. If the BMI criteria are not met, patients (including those who pay privately) must achieve a lower BMI before they are given a referral for specialist fertility treatment (National Women's Health 2021). In addition to investigating cultural and institutional bias around weight norms (Tremellen et al. 2017), Righarts and colleagues (2015) argue that further research is required to determine if the current BMI criteria needs modifying to accommodate to differing body fat compositions among Pacific populations.

There is little research into the experiences of Pacific peoples' access to assisted reproductive technologies in Aotearoa | NZ. Available studies that make reference to Pacific peoples and infertility indicate that inequitable fertility outcomes arise from a combination of factors such as poor access to primary health care, health morbidities associated with low socio-economic status, lack of cultural familiarity with the clinical context, and conflicting socio-cultural values that prevent the disclosure of sexual and reproductive health concerns (Tiatia 2008; Foaese 2017; Righarts et al. 2021). Most women and couples are referred to fertility specialist services by primary health services. For Pacific women who experience barriers to accessing primary health care, as many do, referral for medical fertility treatment may not be sought, or be more difficult to access.

International literature shows that the majority of individuals from Indigenous and ethnic minority groups experience delays and disparities in accessing fertility services (Bendikson et al. 2005; Mascarenhas et al. 2020). In the USA, women from Asian/Pacific Islander, African American and Hispanic backgrounds reported longer durations of infertility and accessed assisted reproductive technologies at a later age compared to white women (Butts 2021). Specifically, African American and Hispanic women found it more difficult to find a physician with whom they felt comfortable and reported it was more difficult to obtain treatment because of their ethnicity (Humphries et al. 2016). In Australia, Aboriginal and Torres Strait Islander women continue to experience greater socio-economic disadvantages than non-Indigenous women when addressing infertility issues and accessing fertility treatment care (Gilbert et al. 2021). Medical help seeking and access to fertility care is similarly compromised for Pacific women in Aotearoa | NZ (Righarts et al. 2021). We explore why in the following discussion.

## Method

The data on which this chapter is based come from a larger qualitative project involving 39 semi-structured interviews conducted by Rhonda, the Principal Investigator, and Edmond, the Pacific lead researcher, documenting individuals' experiences of infertility and access to assisted reproductive technologies in Aotearoa | NZ. Of the interviews undertaken, eight were with Pacific women. The dataset with Pacific women employed a *talanoa* research method to enable Edmond, a self-identified Tongan and Pacific Islander man, to explore sensitivities around infertility in a culturally appropriate way. The term talanoa, which means 'to talk informally, to tell stories or related experiences' (Churchward 1959), describes an open dialogue where people can speak from their hearts. The beauty of talanoa is that researchers are flexible about the direction of the conversation and generous with their time. The conversation ends when the talanoa starts to revisit topics that have already been covered in the discussion (Vaioleti 2006).

Recruitment for the study presented several major challenges. In addition to difficulties recruiting participants from a relatively small population, we were aware that infertility is not often openly discussed in Pacific communities in Aotearoa | NZ. The stigma surrounding infertility and the perceived fear of being exposed as 'infertile' contributes to the silencing of fertility issues for Pacific peoples. We used snowball sampling and word-of-mouth to invite potential interviewees to participate in the study. While it may be uncommon in the Pacific for a man to conduct a talanoa that addresses sensitive issues concerning women, Edmond undertook several preliminary conversations with the participants prior to the formal interview. This was to establish trust, strengthen relationships, and assure participants that that confidentiality was paramount. All study participants have been given pseudonyms in this chapter. The study received research ethics approval from Te Herenga Waka | Victoria University of Wellington and Auckland University of Technology.

Of the eight Pacific women in the study two had successful pregnancies through in vitro fertilisation, two were in the initial stages of fertility treatment, and four had been unable to conceive and were actively considering whether to contact a fertility clinic or not. At the time of the interviews two women were married, five were separated and one was divorced. Five women reported having been diagnosed with either endometriosis or polycystic ovary syndrome. Three women had not yet consulted a doctor to discuss their difficulties conceiving. Of the five who were separated, three participants and the one divorcee attributed their current marital status of being 'single' to their infertility. All eight women were between 35 and 45 years of age. All lived in major Aotearoa | NZ cities. Eight women who participated were of Samoan descent, one woman identified as Tongan and seven were Aotearoa | NZ-born. All participants identified being affiliated with a Pentecostal Christian church.

The talanoa were originally planned to take place face-to-face but because of the COVID-19 epidemic in Aotearoa | NZ, they were conducted online using Zoom. Each talanoa averaged between 45 and 90 minutes and was recorded, with all talanoa being conducted in English. Transcribed transcripts were sent to participants to determine the accuracy and validity of their experiences and insights. Re-listening and re-reading the audio recordings and transcripts respectively were then followed by colour coding. Thematic analysis was conducted manually to identify key themes, and the data were analysed and written up by Edmond and Rhonda.

We begin by examining the infertility experiences of Pacific women using a case study method. Case studies have often been viewed as a useful tool for the preliminary exploratory stage of research projects in surveys and experiments (Crowe et al. 2011), as well as in qualitative research approaches (Stark and Torrance 2005). The key themes presented in the case studies were triangulated using the ongoing talanoa conversations and storying with the Pacific participants involved in this study.

## Findings

Four major themes were identified in the dataset: family expectations; spiritual influence; cultural influence; and fertility treatment aspects of the participants' reproductive journeys. Each theme focuses on the story of one participant. Together, these themes represent intersecting axes of influence, illuminating the various ways participants encountered challenges accessing assisted reproductive technologies.

### *Family expectations – Malu*

Malu was an Aotearoa | NZ-born Samoan woman in her early 40s. Married for over 10 years, Malu and her husband are yet to have children. Malu acknowledges her strong Christian faith, Samoan culture and collective effort of her immediate and extended family, for their sacrifices in leaving Samoa to migrate to Aotearoa |

NZ. Malu has an annual average income of NZD60,000–NZD100,000, therefore making it possible to pay for fertility treatment at a private clinic. Malu has consulted with fertility specialists and has had several unsuccessful attempts with in vitro fertilisation. A very emotional Malu described how she and her husband had reached the embryo transfer stage three times and yet, after each cycle, the transfer was unsuccessful.

Malu, like the majority of study participants, belongs to a 'big Pacific family' that provides her with support, time and space to offload issues about her life, as well as offering prayers and words of encouragement. All the participants acknowledged the role of family in supporting their personal and professional lives, and all contrasted their family of origin to smaller-sized Aotearoa | NZ European families. Each participant reflected on their 'expected' pathway to adulthood that involved secondary school, followed by university, finding a spouse and then having children. Malu described this trajectory as the life plan both she and her parents had in mind for her. Several participants noted the added pressure from their parents (and family) not only to succeed in education and find a good job, but to have children in order to become grandparents. All these expectations and dreams were put on participants without families fully understanding the everyday fertility issues the women faced. Malu shared expectations from her family:

> When I was in university, my cousins and family would talk about how they would want me to get married, I must have a family, must have children, and all of that family stuff. At first, I ignored it and now you reach that stage of almost being expired (age wise), but now I am getting pressure from all my cousins.

Not only do families place expectations on each other, as shared by Malu, but importantly they also play a key role in their health. Pulu and colleagues (2021) note that in Pacific communities families provide much needed and valuable pastoral care and relational support; families also influence health decisions and health seeking behaviours. While study participants agreed with the proverb 'it takes a village to raise a child,' they also shared how this belief amplified the pressure on them to bear children. For Malu and others, this meant that family could not always be relied on to provide the psychosocial support needed to cope with or address infertility. Malu, therefore feared being stigmatised and judged, and rarely shared the burden infertility brought.

Although most Pacific cultures are patrilineal, motherhood plays a key role. In Samoa and Tonga, for example, the primary responsibility of married women is to reproduce progeny to pass down and continue lineages and legacies of the family, and in some cases, the distribution of land. Malu spoke of the importance that bearing children, and then grandchildren, play in Pacific cultures in establishing and securing a person and their family' status within the wider family and community. Labelled the 'infertile child,' Malu felt the weight of constantly attempting to have children. Talking about the perceived failure to fulfil her cultural responsibilities for her husband and his family, she remarked:

> Obviously, everyone looks at you after nine months and then expects you to hold a baby and then 10 years go by and still no rocking lullaby chair. Family is important and blood and all of that kind of stuff, but now it makes it worse because the church and community make comments, [have] opinions, and [make] judgements because of my infertility.

Participants interpreted ongoing difficulties with conception as a sign to get a health check. As a consequence of a health assessment, six women and their partners stopped smoking, reduced their alcohol consumption and focused on healthy eating, regular exercise and creating safe spaces to discuss stress, anxiety and mental health. Several participants commented that this gave them an opportunity to inform their families they were 'trying' their very best to get pregnant. As Malu shared:

> There were a few things that myself had to do and my husband had to do and that was around you know being healthy. So, losing weight, looking at your food, and then for my husband is cutting back on the smoking side of things. So just a few health tips just to get us started … my husband pushed and motivated me to do this, and it was good because there were times where I was down, he would always be there to give me that extra support and motivation.

### *Spiritual influence – Mati*

In her 40s, Mati was a Aotearoa | NZ-born woman of Samoan heritage. Together with her current husband Mati is a strong and devout Christian and is currently attending a church outside the traditional Samoan Methodist church of her parents and family. Religion is central to Pacific identities, with 83% of the Pacific population identifying as religious (Fairbairn-Dunlop and Makisi 2003), and Mati is no exception. With an annual average income of over NZD100,000, Mati has the financial means to afford fertility treatment in private fertility clinics. Mati and her husband have one child conceived through the use of assisted reproductive technologies and are seeking to have more children.

As in much of Pacific life, all of the eight women in this study spoke of fertility – a life event – in spiritual terms, with children viewed as a gift or blessing from God. In the Samoan context, the concept of *feagaiga*, the sacred covenant, has its roots in the principle that women have the gift of producing and nurturing life and, as child-bearers, women share divinity with the pre-Christian gods (Bentham 2008). Consequently, some Pacific women in the study interpreted infertility as 'God's will.' Unlike biomedical explanations of infertility that locate difficulties with conception in terms of individual bodily impairment, the cause of infertility for people of faith is often attributed to 'purposeful intervention' and to 'somebody or something outside the woman (or couple)' (van Balen 2009, p. 37), as was the case with Mati who saw herself as being cursed.

> I married my ex-husband without the blessing of my family or village, which, reflecting about it now, may be a reason why this whole thing took place. It was something that haunted me for years. It could be the reason why I wasn't blessed with a child. Like it could have even been a curse. I guess as a result of not getting their blessing and me running away and getting married, it forced me to go back to Samoa and ask for their apology … not sure if it is a superstitious thing but after getting the blessings from my family in Samoa and then going through in vitro fertilisation a couple of years after, man, I was so shocked that I was pregnant from the treatment and all I can think about is the apology.

Religious beliefs play a central role in making sense of infertility and identifying ways to overcome it. Several participants commented on how often they would be encouraged to pray and regularly attend and contribute to church services and practices to increase their chances of becoming pregnant. Failure to do so would perpetuate their infertility. Mati explained how fertility treatment is perceived as both irrelevant and ineffective if a spiritual connection with God is absent. She shared:

> I remember a year after my marriage where my parents and other members of family would keep dropping comments to me and my husband to maybe pray every day and attend church every Sunday, and even choir practices, and then maybe we could have a child. It was hard to swallow at first, especially for my husband, but then we got over it.

In line with sexual and reproductive health research, studies have shown that young people who have a strong religious affiliation are less likely to initiate or engage in open discussion about sex, and some studies indicate that teenagers who attend religious services frequently are less likely to have any interest in engaging in discussion about sex (Kirby and Lepore 2007). Religious beliefs can therefore hinder discussion about sex, which in turn preclude conversations around fertility and seeking medical advice in relation to assisting reproduction. For some participants then, assisted reproduction was viewed as a blessing to enter a space they envisaged as 'scientific creation,' although doing so went against their views of 'God's creation' and the views of their parents, family and culture. For these participants, the promise of technology gave them a sense of relief that bearing a child could be a reality. As Mati reflected:

> That was the first barrier, and we didn't go beyond that until I was prepared. Like I took counsel from lots of people over many years, to the point where, you know, we're not doing God's work in a different way or anything that way. We're utilizing what he's given us to do … I found myself explaining things in different ways and then I tried to scientifically discuss, which didn't go to plan so, I just got over the questions and was like, if this is God's kind of work you know, let it be, let it be that I do whatever it takes to have children. So, it was hard.

Pacific peoples recognise that religious leaders are important authorities, whose opinions and views can impact people's ideas and practices about health (Bentham 2008; Cammock et al. 2014). It is therefore not surprising that religious leaders would be expected to play an integral part in supporting and encouraging individuals and couples who go through fertility issues. However, none of the participants felt comfortable sharing their fertility challenges with church leaders. When asked why, they noted the smallness of the Pacific community and that church and religious leaders may not have the counselling necessary to provide well informed advice. Furthermore, several participants commented on how church leaders would emphasise the sole importance of focusing on praying, fasting and reading the Bible daily. As Mati remarked:

> Never have and will feel safe nor comfortable in addressing my infertility issues with a religious leader, especially if they are Samoan because of a couple of things. One, they are not trained in the field nor have any understanding and also our community is so small, that I will not be surprised if my family would find out the next day. They will just tell me to pray hard, which I believe they have no idea that I already do so ... they would assume that I am cursed.

### *Cultural influence – Mosi*

In her mid-40s, Mosi was a Aotearoa | NZ-born Samoan. She has an annual average income of NZD60,000–NZD100,000, therefore making it possible to pay for fertility treatment privately. Being married for over five years to her husband, Mosi's experience with assisted reproductive technologies was with her first-born child who was conceived quickly. Mosi's second-born child was conceived without the use of assisted reproductive technology.

In addition to the importance of motherhood in many Pacific cultures, the acceptance of informal adoption within families is thought to reduce the stigma and shame attached with infertility. While none of the participants had adopted children, the majority commented that if they did then family members would encourage them to adopt from the immediate and wider family to ensure that the child has a 'blood connection.' Several participants commented on the perception of fertility treatment as being expensive for Pacific peoples. At the same time, it was agreed that bearing a child is worth all the financial stress and expense associated with the fertility treatment process. As Mosi stated:

> I remember getting slight remarks from my family when they knew we were going through in vitro fertilisation to adopt so and so because she's pregnant and save money and the pain of going through the fertility treatment. I guess I just had to never give up on my faith and trust the science.

Mosi disclosed how she fell in love and got married with her now husband without the blessing of her parents, elders, and wider family. Similar to Mati, Mosi felt like her infertility was the result of not abiding to Samoan culture.

> I went back to Samoa and got their family and village blessing whereas I didn't, and you know, it is a big in Samoan and other Pacific cultures to gain blessings from family and village. Although I gained their blessing later in life, I believe it was too late because I had already hurt them earlier.

Culturally, gaining consent and blessings from parents, grandparents and, at times, other key family members to be married may determine whether a woman is able to bear children or not. Mosi also emphasised the cultural importance of getting permission from elders, in case of support should any marital challenges or issues arise. Born and raised in Aotearoa | NZ, Mosi acknowledged that such cultural pressures may be a cultural shock for other Aotearoa | NZ-born Samoans due to the lack of fully understanding Samoan language and culture. Such challenges could put the reputation of the family, village and Samoan culture at risk, as Mosi pointed out:

> Gaining permission is is like gaining a blessing. It is something that is unwritten in our Samoan culture. It is a must. Not a lot of people value it but when you are immersed in the Samoan culture, it is very important. It is not just marriage; it is a rite of passage for anything you do when you leave the village and every journey.

In Samoan folklore, infertility is highly stigmatised and considered deviant or 'promiscuous' (Walsh et al. 2015, p. 250). In a patriarchal society, it is considered an obligation for Samoan females to have children to carry on and pass down genealogy and land (Bentham, 2008). Culture and religion intersect here, due to the fact that sex which falls short of family formation is decoupled from procreation. As a result, several participants shared how talking openly about infertility and assisted reproductive technologies in Pacific families and communities could demystify infertility as a 'secret stigma' (Greil et al. 2010). Mosi, for instance, remarked that breaking down cultural barriers and normalising informal discussions about sex and reproduction in families is a step in the right direction. She added that there was a need to establish and nurture gender specific spaces for these discourses to take place. In Mosi's view:

> It is important that in order to even be talking about assisted reproductive technologies and even infertility, we [Pacific] need to start addressing sex and making it a norm and not putting a curse that you have sex before marriage, you'll be punished to the extent of not having kids. We [Pacific] just need to keep breaking barriers and allow for safe spaces for girls and couples to share their issues freely without feeling judged and cursed culturally.

### *Fertility treatment services – Moana*

Moana was a Aotearoa | NZ-born Tongan woman in her mid-30s. Throughout the talanoa Moana was emotional, describing how her infertility challenges were the cause of separation from her husband of 10 years. Moana acknowledged the constant support from immediate and extended family members, and at times, words of encouragements with her infertility journey. In terms of annual average income, Moana also earns between NZD60,000 and NZD100,000. Moana has consulted with fertility treatment specialists several times, with one successful attempt with IVF.

Consistent across the talanoa with all interviewees, it was repeatedly reflected that there is a need to raise awareness and education around assisted reproductive technologies. In the only other qualitative study of Pacific women and infertility undertaken in Aotearoa | NZ, Foaese (2017) maintains that education programmes can increase awareness and understanding of assisted reproductive technologies in culturally appropriate and relevant ways for Pacific communities. A key concern for Pacific women in this respect relates to Western ideals around BMI. All the study participants commented on their individual concerns with BMI criteria, self-diagnosing themselves as overweight or obese before going to see a doctor about fertility issues. The women also had ambivalent feelings about the BMI norm as a clinical requirement for accessing fertility treatment. When Moana was informed that her second cycle of in vitro fertilisation had failed, she said:

> I was told 'maybe you should focus on losing weight,' which was something I had done prior, and I knew that because I was trying to eliminate any risks. I was dieting and had dropped a lot of weights to the point where I knew I couldn't go any further and then be told that I need to lose weight, it was like, 'C'mon, I am Tongan.' My mother was like, 'you are looking very fragile after losing a lot of weight,' 'you need to eat' and I was like 'I can't because I have been told that this is probably why it isn't working because I still have to lose weight.'

In Foaese's (2017) study, young Pacific peoples shared that accessing sexual health care services was often associated with the fear that they would be seen by family and church members. Naea (2008) found that Samoan parents who hold traditional values and beliefs need to be educated on the importance of giving and understanding correct sexuality education information. Similar views were shared by participants in this study when accessing fertility treatment centres. Additionally, the Aotearoa | NZ-born Samoan women in the study described how Pacific elders, church officials and community leaders must understand the intricacies of infertility issues and the potential benefits of assisted reproductive technologies. Two participants recommended the value of having this information appropriately distributed within church communities. Moana posited that it would be:

> Very important for churches, particularly our traditional Pacific churches to have information or flyers about how [to] access fertility treatment centres for couples who have been trying [to have children] for years. This will help church leaders understand the struggles that some families may be experiencing.

Pacific populations are overrepresented in socio-economic indicators such as poverty and unemployment (Urale et al. 2019) and are thus more likely to encounter financial barriers accessing fertility treatment unless they qualify for public funding. All study participants knew the high cost of infertility treatment even before making the initial consultation with fertility treatment specialists; such costs are displayed on fertility clinic websites and regularly mentioned in the news media. Despite the fact that participants reported annual average salaries that enabled them to afford their treatment, this may not be the case for the majority of Pacific women in Aotearoa | NZ. Nonetheless, participants from this study highlighted the lack of understanding of financial stresses that come with paying for fertility treatment. Several commented that lack of knowledge about public funding contributed to their initial hesitation to seek information regarding fertility treatment, particularly in vitro fertilisation. Moana remarked:

> Money was definitely an issue for me and that was even before going in and consulting with the clinic because you hear of stories and how difficult and technical everything is making it very expensive. But when I consulted with the specialists, I didn't realise there was a public funding stream for it.

Lack of Pacific fertility treatment specialists was identified as another barrier to getting fertility treatment, making it difficult for Pacific women to feel comfortable and relaxed in the clinic and in interactions with specialists. One participant commented, 'it is hard enough to deal with your condition without doctors not providing a safe environment for you to feel safe.' In addition to observations regarding the lack of Pacific fertility clinic staff, there was criticism about the absence of information on clinic websites in the Pacific language. For participants, these cultural nuances were seen as important ways of making Pacific peoples feel safe and at ease when seeking, understanding and using fertility treatment.

## Discussion

This chapter draws on findings from exploratory research to capture Pacific perspectives on infertility and barriers to accessing assisted reproductive technologies in Aotearoa | NZ. As infertility is a sensitive and invisible topic in Pacific communities, there is a need to educate and increase awareness of fertility treatment services to support Pacific peoples who may struggle with conception. Based on the experiences of Pacific women, we identified four intersecting barriers to accessing assisted reproductive technologies: family expectations; spiritual influences; cultural influences; and fertility treatment service concerns. To help mitigate the problems associated with these issues we make some suggestions based on the talanoa with study participants.

It was suggested by most participants that Pacific families need to be more aware of assisted reproductive technologies and lessen expectations to bear children as this can create stress, anxiety and other mental health issues. Many participants also called for further research and awareness to ensure access to fertility treatment is culturally appropriate. All participants advanced the need for religious leaders to assume a neutral understanding of fertility issues instead of having preconceived ideas and judgements towards Pacific individuals and couples. Several participants recommended that medical and fertility specialists conduct awareness workshops for religious leaders to inform them of assisted reproductive technologies. While these participants recommended Pacific cultural training for fertility treatment specialists, they also sought to address and identify whether there is a culturally specific Pacific understanding of fertility and infertility. They likewise proposed that Pacific families and communities break down cultural barriers to create safe spaces in which to address sensitive issues such as sex and infertility. Some participants recommended the importance of informal social groups to share experiences and insights, which could then empower and encourage others who may go through similar journeys.

It was proposed that a better understanding of treatment techniques such as laparoscopy, intrauterine insemination, donor insemination, surrogate pregnancy arrangements, and gamete donation is needed to improve fertility literacy of Pacific peoples. Furthermore, clinicians and fertility specialists need to be culturally aware of Pacific people's reticence to consult and navigate clinic website resources due to a lack of awareness of the benefits, risks and consequences of fertility treatment procedures. Fertility clinic providers should therefore improve culture and language-concordant care as a step to increase access to assisted reproductive technologies for Pacific communities. Finally, with the majority of the Pacific population in Aotearoa | NZ residing in low socio-economic areas, there is a need to consider fertility treatment services in such locations, and to provide greater availability and accessibility, at lower cost, for women and couples seeking these services in city centres.

## Conclusion

Despite the introduction of assisted reproductive technologies over four decades ago, infertility continues to be a global medical and health issue that affects many individuals and couples. Such technologies offer the promise of hope to transform years of infertility burdens into fertility blessings for those affected, as well as their families and communities. While many factors contribute to the decline of Pacific fertility, there is still a lack of research, awareness and information tailored for Pacific women and couples in relation to fertility treatment in Aotearoa | NZ. A specific focus on Pacific women's infertility in Aotearoa | NZ enhances understanding of this phenomenon but the need remains to further explore infertility from Pacific men's perspective. Men are important in this story; not all causes of infertility relate to women but more importantly, irrespective of where the cause of infertily lies, the inability to reproduce is a shared issue for the couple. While this chapter has focused on infertility among Pacific women in Aotearoa | NZ it does not necessarily speak to Pacific women more broadly in the Pacific, or Pacific women who may seek to travel abroad to neighbouring countries like Aotearoa | NZ and Australia for fertility treatment. Future research into these and related issues is called for.

## Acknowledgements

Thank you to the Pacific women who shared their personal experiences and fertility challenges and the Royal Society NZ Marsden Fund for supporting this research.

## References

Bendikson, K., et al., 2005. Ethnic background and in vitro-fertilisation outcomes. *International Journal of Gynaecology and Obstetrics*, 88 (3), 342–346. doi:10.1016/j.ijgo.2004.11.022

Bentham, E., 2008. *Aspects of Samoan Indigenous spirituality and Christian spirituality and spiritual direction*. Auckland, New Zealand: Spiritual Growth Ministries.

Butts, S., 2021. Health disparities of African Americans in reproductive medicine. *Fertility and Sterility*, 116 (2), 287–291. doi:10.1016/j.fertnstert.2021.06.041

Cammock, R., Derrett, S., and Sopoaga, F., 2014. An assessment of an outcome of injury questionnaire using a Pacific model of health and wellbeing. *New Zealand Medical Journal*, 127 (1388), 32–40.

Churchward, M., 1959. *Tongan dictionary*. London. Oxford University Press.

Crowe, S., et al., 2011. The case study approach. *BMC Medical Research Methodology*, 11 (100), 1–9. doi:10.1186/1471-2288-11-100

ESHRE (European Society of Human Reproductive and Embryology), 2018. *Focus on reproductive*. Grimbergen, Belguim: ESHRE. Available from: www.eshre.eu [Accessed 26 January 2018].

Fairbairn-Dunlop, P. and Makisi, G.S., 2003. *Making our place: Growing up PI in New Zealand*. Palmerston North: Dunmore Press.

Farquhar, C.M. and Gillett, W.R., 2006. Prioritising for fertility treatments—should a high BMI exclude treatment? *BJOG: An International Journal of Obstetrics & Gynaecology*, 113 (10), 1107–1109. doi:10.1111/j.1471-0528.2006.00994.x

Fertility Society of Australia, 2016. Patient information. Available from: http://www.fertilitysociety.com.au/patients-information/ [Accessed 26 January 2018].

Foaese, A., 2017. *Pasifika women's experiences of infertility in Canterbury and Wellington*. Master's thesis, University of Otago, New Zealand.

Gilbert, E., et al., 2021. 'We are only looking at the tip of the iceberg in infertility': Perspectives of health providers about fertility issues and management among Aboriginal and Torres Strait Islander people. *BMC Health Services*, 21 (704), 1–12. doi:10.1186/s12913-021-06714-8

Goodman, L.K., et al., 2020. Reporting assisted reproductive technology success rates on Australian and New Zealand fertility clinic websites. *Australian and New Zealand Journal of Obstetrics and Gynaecology*, 60, 135–140. doi:10.1111/ajo.13126

Greil, A., Slauson-Blevins, K., and McQuillan, J., 2010. The experience of infertility: A review of recent literature. *Sociology of Health and Illness*, 32 (1), 140–162. doi:10.1111/j.1467-9566.2009.01213.x

Humphries, L., et al., 2016. Influence of race and ethnicity on in vitro fertilisation outcomes: Systematic review. *American Journal of Obstetrics and Gynaecology*, 214 (2), 212–217. doi:10.1016/j.ajog.2015.09.002

Institute of Environmental Science and Research Ltd (ESR), 2019. *Sexually transmitted infections in New Zealand: Annual surveillance report 2016*. Porirua, New Zealand. Available from: www.surv.esr.cri.nz [Accessed 6 December 2021].

Kirby, D. and Lepore, G., 2007. *Sexual risk and protective factors: Factors affecting teen sexual behavior, pregnancy, childbearing and sexually transmitted disease: Which are important? Which can you change?* Washington, DC: The National Campaign to Prevent Teen and Unplanned Pregnancy.

Mascarenhas, M., Kulkarni, M., and Balen, A., 2020. Can the ethnic differences in IVF cycle outcome be influenced by the impact of BMI? *Human Fertility*, 24 (4), 275–281. doi:10.1080/14647273.2018.1563915

McQueen, D., et al., 2015. Racial disparities in in vitro fertilisation outcomes. *Fertility and Sterility*, 104 (2), 398–402. doi:10.1016/j.fertnstert.2015.05.012

Meleisea, M. and Schoeffel, P., 1998. Samoan families in New Zealand: The cultural context of change. In: V. Adair and R. Dixon (eds), The family in Aotearoa/*New Zealand*. Auckland, New Zealand: Addison Wesley Longman, 158–178.

Mourad, S., et al., 2019. Measuring patient-centredness in publicly funded fertility care: A New Zealand validation and international comparison of patient-centred questionnaire-infertility. *Australian and New Zealand Journal of Obstetrics and Gynaecology*, 59 (2), 265–271. doi:10.1111/ajo.12869

Naea, M., 2008. *Navigating many worlds: Samoan mothers' views on sexuality education*. Master's thesis, University of Auckland, New Zealand.

National Women's Health, 2021. *Public funding*. Available from: https://nationalwomenshealth.adhb.govt.nz/our-services/fertility/public-funding/ [Accessed 19 October 2021].

Pulu, V., et al., 2021. Investigating principles that underlie frameworks for Pacific health research using a co-design approach: Learnings from a Tongan community-based project. *Pacific Health Dialog*, 21 (7), 399–406. doi:10.26635/phd.2021.115

Righarts, A., et al., 2015. Infertility and outcomes for infertile women in Otago and Southland. *New Zealand Medical Journal*, 128 (1425), 43–53.

Righarts, A., et al., 2021. The burden of infertility in New Zealand: A baseline survey of prevalence and service use. *Australian and New Zealand Journal of Obstetrics and Gynaecology*, 61 (3), 439–447. doi:10.1111/ajo.13323

Stark, S. and Torrance, H., 2005. Case Study. In: B. Somekh and C. Lewin (eds), *Research methods in the social sciences*. London: Sage, 33–40.

Statistics New Zealand, 2019. Parenting and fertility trends in New Zealand: 2018. Stats NZ, 23 October. Available from: https://www.stats.govt.nz/reports/parenting-and-fertility-trends-in-new-zealand-2018 [Accessed 6 December 2021].

Sun, H., et al., 2019. Global, regional, and national prevalence and disability-adjusted life-years for infertility in 195 countries and territories, 1990-2017: Results from a global burden of disease study, 2017. *Aging*, 11 (23), 10952–10991. doi:10.18632/aging.102497

Tiatia, J., 2008. *Pacific cultural competencies: A literature review*. Wellington: Ministry of Health of New Zealand.

Tremellen, K., Wilkinson, D., and Savulescu, J., 2017. Should obese women's access to assisted fertility treatment be limited? A scientific and ethical analysis. *Australian and New Zealand Journal of Obstetrics and Gynaecology*, 57 (5), 569–574. doi:10.1111/ajo.12600

Tupai-Firestone, R., et al., 2016. Understanding Pasifika youth and the obesogenic environment, Auckland and Wellington, New Zealand. *New Zealand Medical Journal*, 129 (1434), 22–35.

Urale, P.W.B., O'Brien, M.A., and Fouché, C.B., 2019. The relationship between ethnicity and fertility in New Zealand. *Kōtuitui: New Zealand Journal of Social Sciences Online*, 14 (1), 80–94. doi:10.1080/1177083X.2018.1534746

Vaioleti, T., 2006. Talanoa research methodology: A developing position on Pacific research. *Waikato Journal of Education*, 12, 21–34. doi:10.15663/wje.v12i1.296

van Balen, F., 2009. Infertility and culture: Explanations, implications and dilemmas. In: L. Culley, N. Hudson, and F. van Rooij (eds), *Marginalized reproduction: Ethnicity, infertility and reproductive technologies*. London: Earthscan, 34–48.

Walsh, M., et al., 2015. Prevalence of *chlamydia trachomatis* infection in Samoan women aged 18 to 29 and assessment of possible risk factors: A community-based study. *Transactions of The Royal Society of Tropical Medicine and Hygiene*, 109 (4), 245–251. doi:10.1093/trstmh/trv014

WHO (World Health Organization), n.d. Infertility. Available from: https://www.who.int/health-topics/infertility [Accessed 1 November 2021].

# 9 Socio-structural influences on young men's experiences of sex, pregnancy and pregnancy prevention in Papua New Guinea

*Herick Aeno,* Elke Mitchell,* Sophie Ase,[1] Richard Nake Trumb, Priscilla Selon Ofi, Angela Kelly-Hanku and Stephen Bell*

## Introduction

Each year approximately 21 million young women aged 15–19 years globally become pregnant, with 12 million of these young women living or giving birth in low- and middle-income countries (WHO 2020). Complications during pregnancy and childbirth remain a leading cause of death for young women in these settings, with the highest risk being to those under 16 years of age (UNFPA et al. 2015; WHO 2020). In Papua New Guinea contraceptive use among young people is low, resulting in the country having one of the highest adolescent fertility rates in Asia and the Pacific (65 births per 1,0000 women aged 15–19 years) (UNFPA et al. 2015).

In Papua New Guinea, unintended pregnancy is more frequent among unmarried women and women who become sexually active at or before 15 years of age (Gupta et al. 2021; Peach et al. 2021). As elsewhere in the Pacific, pregnancy, including antenatal care and contraception, is viewed as a women's issue in Papua New Guinea (see for example, Gupta et al. 2020). In consequence, women and girls have been the focus of much intervention and research. That said, important attempts have been made to include men in some relevant programming and research (see for example, Holmes et al. 2012; Kura et al. 2013; Davis et al. 2018; Gupta et al. 2020). Despite this, little attention has been given to men's experiences of pregnancy, including the socio-structural factors that enhance the risk of unintended pregnancy among young people (Bell et al. 2018). Recognising and valuing the importance of working with young men, and drawing on concepts of vulnerability and sexual agency, this chapter reports on sexually active young men's efforts to prevent unintended pregnancy.

Socio-structural influences on young people's sexual health in low- and middle-income countries are well recognised (see for example, UNFPA et al. 2015; Bell et al. 2018). Recent work has directed attention towards what has been termed a

* Both authors contributed equally to this chapter.

DOI: 10.4324/9781003142072-11

systematic 'structuring of vulnerability' (Aggleton et al. 2006, p. 4) as it relates to unintended sexual health outcomes. Of importance in tackling the effects of this vulnerability is close examination of the factors preventing young people from accessing the information and services they need to prevent unwanted outcomes of sex such as pregnancy. Relevant socio-cultural factors in this respect include lack of accurate information (often the result of parental and community efforts to discourage premarital sex); unequal power relations between young men and women which inhibit communication and negotiation of contraceptive use; and lack of youth-friendly health services. Yet within such constraints, it is important to identify how young people take action to take care of and foster their sexual health and well-being. Doing so may be seen as a form of 'sexual agency,' defined as the 'processes where young people become sexually active and the strategies, actions and negotiations involved in maintaining relationships and navigating broader social expectations' (Bell 2012, p. 284).

Sex is much more than a behavioural act. It is deeply imbued with personal and social meanings and is therefore best understood as a 'practice,' one that is both relational and gendered. Sexual practices involving two or more people are also socially located in ways that influence decisions about engaging in sex; the types of sexual practices engaged in; forming and breaking relationships; the use of contraceptives; seeking sexual and reproductive health care; and, in the case of unplanned pregnancy, the decision to continue with a pregnancy or not. Even if men do not attend antenatal care or assist their wives during childbirth, in Papua New Guinea, strong heteronormative masculinities prevail with men being key decision makers about women's sexual and reproductive health (see for example, Gupta et al. 2020; Eves 2021). To reduce the harm associated with adverse sexual health outcomes and build caring relationships and positive experiences of sex and sexuality for all, programmes require the meaningful engagement of young men. This means not only shifting discourse about men, particularly young men, but also creating space for their participation.

## Methods

Drawing on findings from a larger qualitative study of young people and pregnancy in Papua New Guinea[2], this chapter focuses on data collected from 14 young men, all of whom had had prior sexual experience. At the time of data collection, five participants were 15 years old, seven were 16 years old, and two were 17 years old; 13 had current sexual relationships with one or more girls, and one had a girlfriend with whom he had chosen not to have sex; seven had not yet experienced pregnancy, two were currently experiencing pregnancy and five had previously experienced an induced abortion.

Seven of the young men lived in a small peri-urban town called Kagamuga, close to Mount Hagen in Western Highlands Province, Papua New Guinea's third largest city with approximately 46,000 residents. Kagamuga is served by a primary health care facility that provides maternal and child health services and run by a Papua New Guinean non-governmental organisation. The other young men lived in remote highland villages in Upper Bena, Eastern Highlands Province. The areas include Megabo 1, where four young men lived, and Megabo 2, part of the more remote Wesan area that borders on Madang and Morobe Provinces, where three of them lived. Megabo 1 has basic services including a school, health facility and small trade stores, and is a two-hour drive on a dirt road from Goroka, the provincial capital with c.19,000 residents. Megabo 2 is a village of 250–300 people, not connected by road, and with no basic services, power or mobile phone networks. Dependent on weather conditions, Megabo 2 is a five to eight hour walk across rivers and mountain ranges from Megabo 1.

A semi-structured interview guide was used to access young people's experiences of pregnancy, birth and parenthood; awareness and experience of sexual, reproductive and maternal health services and support; and understandings of community expectations of young people in relation to sex and relationships. Interviews were conducted by four of the authors from the Papua New Guinea Institute of Medical Research (HA, SA, RNT and PO) in a combination of Pidgin and *tok ples* (local language) in audio-private settings perceived as safe by participants. All were audio recorded, transcribed verbatim and translated into English before being coded using inductive techniques to identify recurring themes relating to young men's experiences of pregnancy. All the names associated with quotes in this chapter are pseudonyms; the first time a participant is cited, we provide information of their age and place of residence.

## Socio-structural influences

### *Limited interactions with health workers*

Young men discussed having limited interactions with health workers for sexual health and pregnancy prevention information or services. Most participants in both settings said that health workers did not do community outreach work. Krish (16, Kagamuga) said, 'they don't come,' and Malik (15, Megabo 2) concurred, 'I haven't seen them with my eyes and or heard anything.' Young men provided various reasons for this lack of support. In Kagamuga where there is a large urban clinic, Gary (15, Kagamuga) said that health workers think there is no need to do outreach because the health facility is so close. In contrast, Wilson (16, Megabo 2) said health care workers think young people could go to the hospital in Goroka, a day's travel from Megabo 2, if they wanted to access information or services to prevent pregnancy, but he had never been.

Young men identified a number of factors that inhibited their interactions with health workers. Noel (16 Kagamuga) said that the health education received from them would generally be ignored by *bikhets* (big heads) or self-confident young people who are unwilling to listen and follow instructions. Mondo (17, Megabo 1) said that previous community outreach events were not well attended because community members 'go to their gardens and are busy and only a few come and show their faces.' Other young men described feelings of shame when talking to health workers about sex. Kalen (16, Kagamugua) said, 'because I am not a grown man, I am ashamed to go ask them such questions.' Talking about why young men in his community did not attend community outreach events, Manda (16, Megabo 1) said, 'most times, they are often shy, so they just go and have sex without condoms', rather than ask for them from a health care worker. Despite having already been involved in an unplanned pregnancy (that he had helped terminate using traditional medicine), Manda pointed to the awkwardness of intergenerational conversations about sex and condoms (see Ali-Traill, Chapter 2 and Tu'I'onetoa et al., Chapter 10):

> I usually tell him, 'Please doctor, I need condoms.' That's what I usually say. He sometimes scolds me. … He normally says, 'Hey, what do you want to do?' You know, I often find it difficult to tell him when he asks me … I just say, 'Shh doctor please!' You know, I find it hard to say I want to do such things [have sex].

Despite these barriers, there was a demand for outreach support from these young men, and evidence of resentment that health workers did not support them in their need for information and condoms. Manda said, 'our community health worker doesn't tell us about it and explain there are such things available.' As a result, Manda sometimes takes it on himself to inform other young people. Gary noted, more pointedly,

> The heath care workers are well known to us, but they don't say such things. … They don't tell us what they know, they only keep it to themselves. … They should make awareness and we should at least know some things about having boy/girl relationships and sex, but they don't tell us.

### *Limited sexual education and support from adults*

Beyond the health sector, young men noted only two further sources of adult support regarding sexual health information – formal education in schools, and informal information received from family and elders.

Young men described receiving very rudimentary school education, referring to a subject called 'personal development,' or 'PD.' James (16, Kagamuga), said, 'I was doing my grade eight … we learned how to prevent pregnancy and sicknesses and things like that.' Manda said, 'I first knew about [sex and pregnancy] in class when I was in grade 7, they brought in one book, and we usually read it.' While Noel had learned about condoms from a teacher when he was in grade 5, young men noted the limitations of this learning both in terms of content, but also the timing in young people lives. For example, conceding he had not translated school-based learning into practice but stating he had received the relevant education only after he had started having sex aged 13, and after his girlfriend had become pregnant and returned to her village in a neighbouring province after he refused to marry her, Silan (15, Kagamuga) said,

'I think the teachers need to teach more [about it] because a lot of teenagers are pregnant and are getting married.'

Other community sources of information rarely described what sex was, what the health consequences of having sex might be, or how these could be avoided. In Kagamuga, young people described older male relations advising young men to wait to have sex when married, and to only have children at this time. This was in contrast to parents and elders in Megabo 1 and 2, where the focus of advice and learning was on teaching young men how to prepare for marriage and how to choose the right wife. Boa (15, Megabo 2) reported how his mother told him, 'you must be careful when having relationship with girls. Look at her life, how her parents live, their coffee gardens or properties they have, and [only] then you [should] have a relationship with them.' Manda had received advice to look for evidence of a young woman's *gutpela pasin* (good attitudes and behaviour) as these qualities would lead to a good, problem free, marriage.

### *Becoming ready for marriage and parenthood, and avoiding pre-marital pregnancy*

Young men described strong social expectations to become married and have children, but the advice they received stressed being patient for both until they were ready for adult life. Marriage and parenthood were deemed matters for adults. In Papua New Guinea, pregnancy and having children has inherent value in reproducing culture, strengthening families, and ensuring the longevity of lineages. It is far more than a biological event (see for example, Kelly et al. 2010). Because of this, there was a strong expectation that young people should avoid pre-marital sex and pregnancy. Young men said expectations were placed on young men to be obedient and respect elders' views. Kalen said for example that he was expected to 'obey my parents and live by their rules,' and listen 'to the leaders and don't create trouble.' James described how young men had to 'submit to our parents [wishes],' even if this included 'not permitting' you to have a girlfriend, as explained by Manda.

Perceived readiness for marriage varied among participants. For example, the parents of young men in school expected them to finish their formal education and, where possible, marry educated young women. These expectations were designed to benefit young men as much as their parents. James reported his parents saying, 'after you complete school, marry an educated girl and you will have a name [reputation] in the community.' Manda explained that his parents 'expected me to pass my grade 10 and I did. So, they currently expect me to complete my grade 12 and go to a university.' His parents stressed the importance of education in being ready to support a wife and family more broadly, 'We are a poor family so you must go and at least be on a government payroll [then] we, the family, will get support from you and live.'

Other ways of becoming ready for marriage and children were having a home and livelihood. In the villages of Megabo 1 and 2, doing so showed maturity especially when combined with having an agricultural livelihood sufficient to sustain a wife and children, and being able to pay the bride price needed to secure and formalise a marriage. Blaze (15, Megabo 1) said,

> If I want to get married, I will prepare some things in the coffee, wild betelnut or red pandanus gardens. We are village people, and we earn money from these things. We normally prepare those and then you are now ready to get married. We also sort out pigs. We normally look after pigs until they are matured, and parents normally observe and say, 'This boy has now changed. He will get married.'

Young men in these villages were aware that a future wife would also have expectations. Allan (16, Megabo 1) said, 'When you want to marry a woman, you must build a house … buy plates and cups, spoons, saucepans, mattresses, pillows and blankets,' and 'make gardens, coffee gardens and plant long-lasting things' and 'build your toilet.' Once these preparations had been made, Allan said, 'You will sweet talk your wife and she will come.' But both Allan and Mando commented that if women came and saw none of these objects in the house or the garden for income generation and food, they would just leave. Similar preparations for marriage and parenthood were mentioned in Kagamuga. However, given the economic opportunities associated with Kagamuga's proximity to Mount Hagen, young men living there referred to the importance of having salaried employment rather than an agricultural income. Regardless of these differences, marriage and preparation for marriage in young men's narratives was synonymous with timely pregnancy and parenthood. Pregnancy and parenthood outside of these parameters was deeply shameful.

### *Consequences of becoming pregnant too soon*

Young men described the emotional challenges they faced when a girlfriend became pregnant outside of marriage. When Wilson was told by others his girlfriend was pregnant, he recalled 'I had this thought [about what people might say], 'Hey he is just a young boy, and he is married and has a child' and I was a little bit scared' Ashamed his girlfriend was pregnant Mando 'hid' the news, saying, 'I didn't want [my parents] to know.' So overwhelmed and stressed by hearing the girl he had had sex with several months earlier was pregnant, James said, 'All my strength was gone, I was also thinking of schooling, I found it difficult, I was scared … everyone scolded me and really hated me.' As a result, he stayed at home, feeling ashamed of getting a girl he did not want to marry pregnant and his parents' withdrawal of support for his school fees.

In the case of an unanticipated pregnancy, young men noted a change in their social relationships with others. They became the centre of community gossip that disparaged them for being involved in community life, an important difference from early research on unplanned pregnancy among young people in a similar geographical area in the country that showed such gossip was only targeted at the girls (Kelly et al. 2010). Jason (17, Kagamuga) described community feelings of 'pity' towards young parents, and how friends 'will make fun of me and will gossip about me.' Boa said,

> they usually say, 'He is a little boy but he has a child' ... They don't usually do good to them ... and when they go home, they also don't speak to them well.

Manda said that young men with a child are called, 'little fathers.' Kalen explained how community members 'say that, "This boy and girl are very young and how did they do that," like it's a deed of immoral behaviour.'

Young men spoke often about the responses and reactions from families linked to their 'disobedience' and having brought shame on the family. Malik and Manda described being 'beaten' and 'scolded' by their parents, while James and Noel said that others would feel and show 'hatred' towards them. Gary said his parents

> ... would reject and forsake me. They would hate and reject me. They will not have a good relationship with me ... They will be angry, they won't be happy when giving me something, they will speak harshly to me.

The consequences of losing family support when a pregnancy occurred was very real. James reflected on what happened to him after his girlfriend became pregnant, 'No they did not support me. I did the thing that they really hated.' Krish said,

> In the past we benefit from our parents. We looked to our parents for food and help. As it is now [when one is pregnant or has a child], we have to work and look for our own food. Parents sometimes are not interested in providing us food and money.

When his mother found him at home with a girl for the second time, Silan described how she 'took me and locked me up in jail [police cell] ... she was angry with me!' but later she let him go and did not bring charges. James explained his family were 'mad' with him due to the money they had invested – and now wasted – on his education when at the age of 15 years, he got a girl pregnant.

In both town and village settings, young men described the difficult lives they observed in other young people who have children too young. Allan said, 'I usually feel sad for them. They live with [the] dirt.' Gary said,

> They ruined their education, they find it difficult to build houses, possess a piece of land, plant a little food garden and feed their wives. Because they find it difficult to feed their wives, they often quarrel with their families ... They are young men who depend on their parents again ... They often need money to wash their clothes, but they find it difficult to access money.

Other consequences spoke to how the issue of pregnancy had to be resolved in the absence of marriage, including the need to compensate the family of the pregnant girl for having 'spoiled her name,' as James described. This likely meant that no other man would want to marry her, her value in terms of bride price was significantly reduced, and her ability to complete school was compromised as pregnant students are routinely expelled from school in Papua New Guinea.

## Constrained sexual agency

### *Young men's hidden sexual experiences*

Given the influences described above, young men felt compelled to make sure their sexual relationships were discreet, as illustrated by Jason who said, 'secretly we befriend them [girls in the community] and lie to our parents.' For some, meet ups with young women for sex occurred during the night. Gary elaborated on the privacy that night-time could afford:

> We tell stories, stay together, walk around at night … We often do such, chat and walk around … I went to her house and called her. … I told her to come, and she came. We sat under a tree, chatted … I hugged her and kissed her, and we did all sorts of things.

Other young men used relatives' vacant houses or invited their girlfriends to their homes when no-one is there. Remembering the first girl he ever had sex with, James said he and a girl had agreed to meet at school late in the afternoon, and had sex in an empty classroom. Silan also spoke of having had sex at school in the classroom at night during a school dance.

These private arrangements to meet and have sex were negotiated between young women and men themselves, without support, or through trusted peers. Highlighting the role of technology in facilitating sexual encounters, James shared that mobile phone texts such as 'please call me,' were used as code to indicate when it was safe to meet for sex. Krish described making arrangements to see one of his girlfriends. Another girl 'takes our messages to her and back to me … she is one of her sisters. She goes and tells her that I am waiting. I go and wait …'

Manda' sexual initiation was facilitated by one of his male friends:

> I was 14 and the first time was just down by the river where [her] house is. A boy arranged it and a girl and I came and slept (had sex) there … [the girl] told the boy, 'sshh … I like your brother (male friend).' The boy and I are mutual friends, so he came and informed me, and I also accepted. We stayed for a week or two and then we came straight to the house [to have sex].

Other young men, including Boa, Malik, Silan and Kalen, described meeting girls at community events such as sports games and dances, where there was sometimes alcohol.

When alcohol was consumed, sex was described as more likely to occur, usually in the absence of short-acting contraception such as condoms. Gary explained,

> when young men are drunk, their desire for sex arises so they often take their girlfriends, have sex with them and make them pregnant. It is only under the influence of alcohol they do such things.

Constrained as it may be, keeping relationships hidden from adults is a form of sexual agency. In these contexts, young men and women chose to engage in sex and relationships but did so in ways that navigated the social expectation that sex should wait until marriage and avoided the consequences arising from sexual activities becoming public knowledge. In contexts where sexual relationships occur in the absence of education about pregnancy prevention, and lack of support from health workers to access short-acting or long-acting reversible contraception, the need to keep relationships secret means that young people are incredibly vulnerable to unwanted pregnancy. In this kind of situation, parents, community leader, health workers and other adults bear some of the responsibility for young people's vulnerability.

### *Pregnancy prevention strategies*

When socio-structural factors limit access to sex and sexuality education for young people, inhibit their interactions with health workers, and constrain supportive networks with informed peers and adults, gaps in young men's understandings about sex, pregnancy and pregnancy prevention strategies are inevitable.

Young men in both the town and village settings described being surprised they could get a girl pregnant. Manda described having sex as 'a pleasurable thing,' but when they continued having sex for fun and the girl became pregnant, he said, 'we were confused that she is now pregnant.' More worryingly, Boa, Wilson and Blaze in Megabo 1 and 2 reported knowing nothing about these issues. The following exchange between the interviewer and Boa illustrates the gaps:

| | |
|---|---|
| *Interviewer:* | All those girls that you slept with, did you do things to prevent them from falling pregnant? |
| *Boa:* | No. |
| *Interviewer:* | Did you use some things? |
| *Boa:* | No. |
| *Interviewer:* | Do you get scared of making them pregnant? |
| *Boa:* | Mmm (Agrees) |
| *Interviewer:* | Have you heard about some things that prevent women from falling pregnant? |
| *Boa:* | No. |

*Interviewer:* When you were in school did some people tell you that if you do these then girl would not fall pregnant?
*Boa:* No.
*Interviewer:* When you were at the village, did some boys tell you such?
*Boa:* No, they didn't.
*Interviewer:* Did some family or some people tell you that if you follow this method, you won't make a girl pregnant?
*Boa:* No.
*Interviewer:* Okay, so you don't have any knowledge how to prevent girls from falling pregnant?
*Boa:* Mmm (Agrees).
*Interviewer:* Have you heard from older boys saying "we usually do that and then girls don't get pregnant"?
*Boa:* No, they haven't told me.

Other participants mentioned the calendar or rhythm method, withdrawal and condoms as ways of preventing pregnancy. However, their understanding and use of these strategies was inconsistent. Silan, Jason, Mando and Manda referred to the calendar method. According to Silan, girls say,

> you can have sex with us when we are having our menstruation or just after we have our menstruation. Don't have sex with us when we have not yet had our menstruation.

But he also added 'they don't usually explain to me. They just say that,' indicating lack of a shared understanding between sexual partners of how the strategy might work. That one of Silan's girlfriends conceived, and later terminated the pregnancy, shows that while young people might use this method, it is not successful in preventing pregnancy. Mondo shared,

> I asked her [about her dates]. If she said it was her wrong time, I wouldn't have had sex with her, but she said, 'Yes, I am free.' I went on top of her and hey! I was confused [she got pregnant]!

And Manda alluded to distrust in his relationship as well:

> I asked [her], 'is the date of your monthly period close by?' I ask them and they said 'no, my monthly period has already passed.' And so we had unprotected sex few times … I ask them but you know sometimes they lie. They lie and say 'shh our period has [passed]' and then they fall pregnant.

Withdrawal was a method commonly discussed by young men in Kagamuga. It had been learned about through peer networks, as well as in school. Silan described his experience as follows:

> I didn't ejaculate in her when I wanted to release. I took it out [ejaculated outside] … I don't normally release on their bodies … [I learned] from my teacher and I saw it in the PD book which the grade 8s normally use … The book said, 'if a lady is 10 years and above, she would still be pregnant even if a small sperm touches her. So, men must be careful.' I saw it and thought, 'I will not release sperm into her … My seniors told me … They normally say, 'don't release your sperm in her if you go around with a woman and have sex with her. Take it out and spray it outside wherever you are.'

Others young men, like Krish, described relying on this method,

> the older boys told me that you are about to come you must pull out of her and ejaculate outside, do not come inside her vagina because it can fertilise an egg and a baby can form.

Condoms were mentioned by young men in both settings, and were perceived as appropriate for use before marriage. Gary and James knew about condoms, but did not know how to use them. Others too knew about condoms and where to obtain them but did not use them. Kalen said,

> the boys normally say you must use condoms but that time … [but] we didn't plan for it and we just went, conversed for a while and had sex so we did not think of using a condom.

Only two participants reported using condoms with their girlfriends. Noel used condoms because, 'I don't want to spoil her reputation.' Manda reported using condoms when it was not safe with the calendar method, although not every time.

Other pregnancy prevention techniques were mentioned, but less frequently so. Three young men in Megabo 1 and 2 described abstaining from sex. Having already got one girlfriend pregnant, Mondo was planning to continue to abstain from sex until he was married. Wilson described just having hugs rather than sex. Two young men described having sex just once to reduce the chance of pregnancy. Gary said, 'I had sex for about 10 minutes, felt satisfied and stood up. I thought I might make her pregnant if I had sex several rounds and for an extended time.'

Other than condoms, only Noel and Manda referred to biomedical forms of contraception. Noel said that,

> some girls go to the hospital and see the nurses, and the nurses give them some medicine to take and when they sleep [have sex] with men, they don't get pregnant.

He did not know any more than this and had not discussed the issue with his girlfriend. Manda on the other hand had a fuller understanding of different contraceptive methods including the oral contraceptive pill, tubal litigation and vasectomy based on what he had learned at school.

On balance, strategies to prevent pregnancy were reasonably well known about, although not always accurately informed, indicative of the agency young men exhibited in finding out about sex in a context of serious constraint. Sharing information in relationships, through peer groups, and in communication with adults in school or the community were forms of interpersonal agency aimed at preventing the occurrence of unwanted pregnancy. Importantly, throughout the study and in both contexts young men recognised the importance of pregnancy prevention but were thwarted in their efforts to practise it by the structured vulnerability created by lack of access to accurate information and the difficulty of accessing supportive health services.

## Concluding thoughts

Contrary to stereotypical portrayals of young men as uncaring and irresponsible, young men in this study were keenly aware of factors influencing their experiences of sex and pregnancy prevention. These included lack of access to youth-friendly, non-judgemental reproductive and maternal health services; lack of conversation between parents and children about young people's desires and practices; lack of sex and sexuality education to fill in knowledge and information gaps about pregnancy prevention options; difficulties talking with sexual partners about pregnancy prevention; and limited connections to well-informed social networks to support evidence informed sexual practices.

While constrained by these factors, young men in the Papua New Guinea highland communities where this study took place demonstrated agency within their sexual relationships and with peers and adults. Reputation management, both for themselves and for others, underpinned many of their actions. For example, young men engaged in sex in secret to avoid the social and family consequences of pre-marital relationships becoming public knowledge. Some also tried to limit the chance of early pregnancy for the benefit of their own futures, for the reputation of girls they were sexually involved with and for the reputation of their families. Given young men's personal experiences of pregnancy, the limits to their understanding of pregnancy prevention options, and their ability to access the health resources needed, the socio-structural constraints on their ability to prevent pregnancy were only too clear.

It is disheartening to note that similar issues have been identified in youth-focused research for many years (see for example, Aggleton et al. 2006; Harrison 2008; Kelly et al. 2010; McMillan and Worth 2011; Bell 2012; UNFPA et al. 2015; Bell et al. 2018). In too many settings, young people remain constrained to protect their sexual and reproductive health in circumstances that are not of their own making. Despite this, our findings point to significant opportunities.

Young men in this study tries to use the information available – however inaccurate, limited or misconceived – in ways to prevent pregnancy from taking place. What they lacked was good quality school-based education about gender, sex and sexuality together with access to youth-friendly sexual and reproductive health services where they (and their partners) could learn about and access modern forms of short- and long-acting reversible contraception from health-care workers capable of engaging with and meeting young people's needs. But by themselves good-quality school education and youth-friendly services are not enough. Across Papua New Guinea and the Pacific young people are raised in and by communities, not by isolated nuclear families. Young people are exposed to new knowledge and ideas at a rapid pace, often much faster than their elders, and work must focus on bridging this divide so that the knowledge that parents and other adults share with young people is done so in ways that recognises and responds to the current realities experienced by young people.

The anthropologist Kathy Lepani (2005 p. 19) once said in relation to HIV that 'talk remains the most tangible resource' in settings like Papua New Guinea. While the ideas and messages shared in such talk may vary between peers, young people and health care workers, and young people, parents and trusted adults in the communities, the ability to converse safely and respectfully with others, to explore and critically examine information and misconceptions, and to be supported to make safe, informed and thoughtful choices is paramount. Intergenerational conversations between young men and their parents and other adults in the community must be more of a focus in future programmes.

That young men in our study were able to talk so seriously about their experiences reiterates calls for the future planning and delivery of sex and sexuality education programmes, and sexual, reproductive and maternal health services, to be carried out in partnership with young people. Young men, as we have argued throughout this chapter need to be intimately involved in these conversations about matters that, while of fundamental importance to women, are intimately relational in nature.

## Notes

1 Sophie Ase was the project coordinator for the study from which this data is drawn, but sadly died in 2020 before the study was completed. We dedicate this chapter to her memory.

2 The study received ethics approval from the Papua New Guinea Institute of Medical Research, the Government of Papua New Guinea's Medical Research Advisory Committee, and Human Research Ethics Committee of UNSW Sydney. Informed written consent was gained from all participants.

## References

Aggleton, P., Ball, A., and Mane, P., 2006. Introduction. In: P. Aggleton, A. Ball, and P. Mane (eds), *Sex, drugs and young people*. London: Routledge, 1–9.

Bell, S., 2012. Young people and sexual agency in rural Uganda. *Culture, Health & Sexuality*, 14 (3), 283–296. doi:10.1080/13691058.2011.635808

Bell, S., et al., 2018. Youth-centred research to help prevent and mitigate the adverse health and social impacts of pregnancy amongst young Papua New Guineans. *Reproductive Health Matters*, 26 (54), 5–12. doi:10.1080/09688080.2018.1512297

Davis, J., et al., 2018 Expectant fathers' participation in antenatal care services in Papua New Guinea: A qualitative inquiry. *BMC Pregnancy and Childbirth*, 18, 138. doi:10.1186/s12884-018-1759-4

Eves, R., 2021. Male intimate partner sexual and reproductive coercion in highlands Papua New Guinea. *Pacific Journal of Reproductive Health*, 1 (13), 667–674.

Gupta, S., et al., 2020. Community attitudes and gendered influences on decision making around contraceptive implant use in rural Papua New Guinea. *Reproductive Health*, 17, 136. doi:10.1186/s12978-020-00985-w

Gupta, S., et al., 2021. Fertility preferences, contraceptive use, and the unmet need for contraception in Papua New Guinea: Key findings from 1996 to 2016. *Asia Pacific Journal of Public Health*, 33 (6-7), 780–783. doi:10.1177%2F10105395211034299

Harrison, A., 2008. Hidden love: Sexual ideologies and relationship ideals among rural South African adolescents in the context of HIV/AIDS. *Culture, Health & Sexuality*, 10 (2), 175–189. doi:10.1080/13691050701775068

Holmes, W., et al., 2012. 'Because it is a joyful thing to carry a baby': Involving men in reproductive, maternal and newborn health in East New Britain, Papua New Guinea. *Papua New Guinea Medical Journal*, 55 (1/4), 24–34.

Kelly, A., et al., 2010. Gendered talk about sex, sexual relationships and HIV among young people in Papua New Guinea. *Culture, Health & Sexuality*, 12 (3), 221–232, doi:10.1080/13691050903181107

Kura, S., Vince, J., and Crouch-Chivers, P., 2013. Male involvement in sexual and reproductive health in the Mendi District, Southern Highlands Province of Papua New Guinea: A descriptive study. *Reproductive Health* 10, 46. doi:10.1186/1742-4755-10-46

Lepani, K., 2005. 'Everything has come up to the open space': Talking about sex in an epidemic. Working Paper #15. Canberra: Gender Relations Centre, Research School of Pacific and Asian Studies, Australian National University.

McMillan, K.E. and Worth, H., 2011. The impact of socio-cultural context on young people's condom use: Evidence from two Pacific Island countries. *Culture, Health & Sexuality*, 13 (3), 313–326. doi:10.1080/13691058.2010.529945

Peach, E., et al., 2021. Risk factors and knowledge associated with high unintended pregnancy rates and low family planning use among pregnant women in Papua New Guinea. *Scientific Reports*, 11 (1), 1222. doi:10.1038/s41598-020-79103-6

UNFPA, UNESCO, and WHO, 2015. *Sexual and reproductive health of young people in Asia and the Pacific: A review of issues, policies and programmes*. Bangkok: UNFPA.

WHO, 2020. Adolescent pregnancy fact sheet. *World Health Organization* [online]. Available from: https://www.who.int/news-room/fact-sheets/detail/adolescent-pregnancy [Accessed 20 July 2022].

# 10 *Fofola e fala ka e talanoa e kāinga* (roll out the mat so that the family can talk): Unplanned pregnancy and support for young women and girls in Tonga

*Telusa Tu'i'onetoa,* Hilary Gorman,**
*Karen McMillan and Christine Linhart*

> My mother noticed there was something different and asked if anything had happened. But I lied to her and said no. My mum didn't believe me because she saw I was different, so she spoke to her cousin at the hospital and arranged for me to be seen, and we found I was five months pregnant... My boyfriend had blocked me on Facebook when he found out about my pregnancy. He got what he wanted [long sigh]. His family does not know anything about me and the baby. But I'm okay with that ... my boyfriend told me to get rid of it because he doesn't want to look after it and raise it. But I told him that I will take care of the baby and he can leave, and I will have no problem finding a father figure for my baby. So, he verbally abused me and left, and I cried because now I know he only used me, he never loved me ... My whole pregnancy was very hard and painful because my heart was broken, my boyfriend hurt me a lot ... I haven't seen my boyfriend ever since [I was pregnant]. And his family doesn't acknowledge me and the baby.
>
> (Angela, pregnant at 16 years, Tongatapu)

## Introduction

Pregnancy, childbirth and motherhood can be transformative life events, often influenced and defined by the sociocultural contexts in which they occur (Reed et al. 2017). For many women, motherhood is a positive experience that gives a sense of purpose with feelings of intense happiness through bonding with the newborn child (Reed et al. 2017). Pacific societies place high value on motherhood, and children are traditionally valued for their contribution to the family as a source of social support and the labour roles they support within the family (Reed et al. 2017; White et al. 2018b).

However, the experience of pregnancy and prospect of motherhood is often not a positive one for young Pacific women and girls who experience an unplanned pregnancy: they tend to react with denial, and fear the social consequences of sharing

* Both authors equally contributed to this chapter.

DOI: 10.4324/9781003142072-12

their pregnancy with their male partner, family and community (Kelly et al. 2010; Bell et al. 2018; White et al. 2018b). In addition, unplanned pregnancy is often a barrier to completion of high school education and opportunities for further education (UNFPA 2013; White et al. 2018b), and as such is considered to negatively impact on the future economic and social prospects of the young mothers.

Bell and Aggleton (2013) note two broad sets of factors that contribute to unplanned pregnancy: individual risks, characterised by an individual's knowledge and behaviour; and societal vulnerability, characterised by socio-cultural, economic, political and legal factors which either facilitate or constrain an individuals' chances of becoming pregnant. Social influences such as age-related expectations and gender social norms, produced and reproduced by both adults and young people, can be used ' … as a lens through which to analyse the broader consequences of young people's relationships, and the influence of social context on sexual practices and outcomes' (Bell and Aggleton 2013, p. 103).

Young women in the Pacific navigate sexual and reproductive decision-making in increasingly complex social and cultural contexts, and these realities can only be adequately grasped through investigation of the lived experiences and consideration of the perspectives of the young women and girls themselves. Angela's[1] narrative above signals to several of the kinds of problems highlighted in recent research with young women who face unplanned pregnancy in Tonga, and it is that data we wish to focus on in this chapter. The young women's stories elucidate points of tension between traditional social norms and the lived realities of sexual and reproductive health for young women in modern-day Tonga; a social context wherein traditional values and norms around young womanhood rub up against the proliferation of social media, civil society organisations advocating for gender equality and broader processes of economic and social development.

The chapter is grounded in data from qualitative in-depth interviews that were undertaken in Tonga in 2019 as part of a study that investigated the lived experiences of unplanned pregnancy among young women and girls. The chapter firstly presents a general overview of unplanned pregnancy among young women and girls in the Pacific and Tonga, and presents some of the findings from the Tonga study. Findings clearly demonstrate a lack of reliable and consistent sexual and reproductive health information for young women and girls in Tonga, as well as a lack of support mechanisms that might help them negotiate the landscape of gender and sexual relations in a locally appropriate way. Thus, the subsequent discussion considers the practice of *talanoa*[2] and poses the potential for utilising or adapting talanoa in a manner that maintains its cultural integrity, in order to better include young women and address their needs around sex and relationship information, and sexual and reproductive health decision-making.

## Unplanned pregnancy among young women and girls in the Pacific

Unplanned pregnancy is driven by structural factors such as gender relations that constrain young women's agency with their male partners, as well as social, cultural and religious norms (Bell et al. 2018). In most Pacific societies social, cultural and religious norms promote the ideal that young unmarried women are to refrain from having sex before marriage, and in an effort to try and uphold these ideals young women tend to be subject to community surveillance and moral judgement (Butt and Munro 2007; Kelly et al. 2010; White et al. 2018b; Mitchell and Bennett 2020). Yet, adolescent fertility rates are high in most Pacific Island countries compared to Pacific rim countries such as Australia and New Zealand (Sorchik et al. 2019; Linhart et al. 2020).

There is limited research focused on the experiences of young women and girls who face unplanned pregnancy in Pacific Island countries. Research on the subjective experiences of unplanned pregnancy among young women in the Cook Islands highlights low levels of knowledge and inconsistent use of contraceptives (White et al. 2018a). Upon learning of their pregnancy, young Cook Islander women reacted with denial and fear of the social stigma associated with their unplanned pregnancy, and many considered abortion but had no local access to abortion services. Upon becoming mothers, they had more positive feelings and received support from their families, but some also described how they struggled with motherhood, especially taking care of their child, and reflected that they wished they had delayed their pregnancy until they were older and able to achieve other life aspirations (White et al. 2018b).

Young women tend to be blamed for unplanned pregnancies much more than their male partners (Bell et al. 2018). A study on perceptions of sexual risk among young heterosexual iTaukei women attending university in Suva, Fiji, found that premarital pregnancy was considered a significant risk due to the potential impact it could have on reputations, family dynamics, education and future romantic relationships (Mitchell and Bennett 2020). In the Fijian context, gender norms determine that with premarital pregnancy there is a much greater risk to the young women's reputation than that of their male partner, and that men as decision-makers determine if a condom is used (Mitchell and Bennett 2020). Similarly, in Papua New Guinea, the shame surrounding premarital pregnancy, and gossip that focuses on the young mothers rather than their male partners, directs the blame for unplanned pregnancy on young women (Kelly et al. 2010).

Globally, in many countries there are taboos around youth sexuality. In the Pacific, traditional social norms strongly influence knowledge and practices around sexual and reproductive health and can be a barrier to accessing sexual and reproductive health services (Bell et al. 2018; O'Connor 2018). In Vanuatu, socio-cultural norms and taboos are the most significant barrier to youth accessing sexual and reproductive health services (Kennedy et al. 2014). Information for young people has tended to focus on sexually transmissible infections (STI) and HIV, while young ni-Vanuatu indicated a preference for more information about pregnancy, condom use, puberty, sexuality and relationships (Kennedy et al. 2014). Similarly, research among young Cook Islanders found that they had little knowledge of pregnancy and prevention of STI, and that they want knowledge and communication skills, particularly about contraception and pregnancy, to enhance their understanding and decision-making in their relationships (Futter-Puati 2017). Recent Fijian data highlighted the role of emotions in sexual and reproductive decision-making among young people, calling for greater attention to the subjective views and understandings of young people themselves, and to the socio-cultural and structural environments that shape them (O'Connor et al. 2018).

In Tonga, as in other parts of the Pacific, gender norms, power dynamics and taboos influence young women's behaviours and relationships (McMillan 2011; McMillan and Worth 2011). Discussion of sexual and reproductive health, domestic violence and gender issues in school, churches and the media are resisted (Austin 2013). Qualitative research focused on condom use among young people in Tonga found that condoms are associated with social transgression (McMillan 2011). Condoms were simultaneously noted as potentially reducing individual risk by preventing unplanned pregnancy before marriage and thus saving damage to one's reputation, but were also a social risk in that accessing and possessing condoms shows the intention to have sex, which if discovered would result in gossip, shame and reputational damage to the individual and their family, especially for young women as it detracts from the ideal of feminine modesty (McMillan 2011). However, a few young men and women participants thwarted the norms and embraced the use of condoms (McMillan 2011). Consideration of the role of identity, culture and tradition, and shifting wider community attitudes, is essential to the account of individual behaviour when it comes to condom use and other aspects of sexual and reproductive health (McMillan and Worth 2011).

## Tonga: social norms in a modern-day Polynesian kingdom

The Kingdom of Tonga is a group of Polynesian islands with an estimated population of around 100,000 people (Tonga Statistics Department 2021). Tongan society identifies as being staunchly Christian and as politically and culturally independent. It is a highly stratified society and is organised in traditional social classes. At the top of the social structure is the King and the royal household; followed by the nobles; and at the bottom are the commoners.

Tonga's social structure is underpinned by traditional values of *anga fakatokilalo/loto tō* (humility), *tauhivaha'a /vā* (reciprocity) and *mamahi'i me'a* (loyalty), grounded on *'ofa* (love) (Vaioleti 2006). *Faka'apa'apa* (respect) is a core value in the family and society. Elders are respected and accredited as voices of wisdom. Young Tongans are expected to demonstrate respect, humility, and love for their parents. Duty to community, conformity to traditional femininity and acquiescence to parental values require young women to abstain from sex until marriage (McMillan and Worth 2011).

Tonga places high value on education, as demonstrated through the literacy rate of 99.4% (99.3% for males and 99.5% for females) among 15–24 year olds in 2018 (UNESCO 2022). The ideal life progression in Tonga is understood as one that conforms to a sequence: obtaining an education, getting a job, marrying a heterosexual partner and creating a family. Pregnancy before marriage defies Tongan social ideals.

The fertility rate of young women and girls aged 15–19 years in Tonga was estimated to be 30 births per 1,000 population during 2014–2019, and was slightly higher in rural areas at 32 per 1,000 than in urban areas at 25 per 1,000 (Tonga Statistics Department 2020). Abortion is illegal in Tonga, but there are a limited number of cases reported of women presenting to health centres for post abortion care (UNFPA 2015). Data collected in 2019 on sexual behaviours and practices indicate that in Tonga 25% of young women and girls and 71% of young men and boys between the ages of 15–24 years had sex in the previous 12 months with a non-marital and non-cohabitating partner; and 15% of young women and girls and 25% of young men and boys used a condom during their last sexual intercourse (Tonga Statistics Department 2020).

## Adolescent unplanned pregnancy study

In July 2019 qualitative interview data was collected in Tonga as part of a larger three-country Pacific study that sought to understand the context and realities of young women and girls who experienced unplanned pregnancy and motherhood in Tonga (Linhart et al. 2020), Vanuatu (McMillan et al. 2020) and Chuuk State in the Federated States of Micronesia (McMillan et al. 2020).[3] Qualitative in-depth face-to-face interviews were conducted with young women and girls aged 16 to 19 years who had experienced an unplanned pregnancy. In acknowledgement of the ongoing cultural importance and use of traditional medicines in many Pacific countries, the study also included enquiries into traditional as well as contemporary means of fertility control, and interviews were conducted with grandmothers or older women aged 50 years and above who were willing to share their knowledge on this topic.

Participants were recruited through convenience and snowball sampling with the assistance of the Talitha Project and the Tonga Family Health Association. Four local research assistants received intensive training and were engaged to work with the research team. In total, 26 face-to-face interviews and one focus group discussion were conducted. Interviews were conducted across three of the main island groups of Tonga: Tongatapu (six interviews with 16–19-year-olds; two interviews with grandmothers or women over 50); Vava'u (six interviews with 16–19-year-olds; seven interviews with grandmothers or women over 50); and Ha'apai (three interviews with 16–19-year-olds; two interviews with grandmothers or women over 50; and one focus group was held with four women over 50). Only one focus group was conducted with grandmothers and older women as they preferred to be interviewed privately. The majority of interviews were conducted in Tongan, with a smaller number conducted in English. All interviews conducted in Tongan were translated into English by a native Tongan speaker fluent in English. Those translations were then checked against the original audio files and verified by a second translator. Pseudonyms have been used to protect the participants' identities. Ethical approval to undertake the study in Tonga was obtained from the Tongan Government and the UNSW Human Subjects Ethics Committee.

## Findings: young women's experiences of unplanned pregnancy

### *Knowledge and access to contraceptives*

Knowledge of sexual and reproductive health was low among this group of young women and girls. Most interviewees were aware of becoming pregnant from engaging in unprotected sex, but did not think that they would become pregnant when they were having unprotected sex. Sources of reliable information about sexual and reproductive health and contraception were limited, with many participants stating that the only things they knew about these topics were what they had seen on Facebook, on YouTube and in movies, which can be inaccurate, misunderstood and portray negative relationship dynamics, including violence against women.

Of the participants who did mention the use of contraception (almost exclusively condoms), its application was inconsistent and at the sole discretion of their male partner. The young women and girls did not mention having any role in negotiating the use of contraception:

> I never knew anything. It was him who usually got those condoms and I don't know where he bought it from or anything. He bought it but he never wanted to use it ... when he's mad, he's going to do it, like he's not going to use a condom.
>
> (Fran, pregnant at 17, Tongatapu)

> When we were dating, he used to come with things like that [condoms] ... He told me it's for protection but after a time we didn't use the condom anymore, maybe that is why I developed this problem. When I got pregnant and I told him, he told me he got me pregnant on purpose in case I have another man.
>
> (Debra, pregnant at 17, Tongatapu)

Their experiences demonstrate the gendered dynamics in relationships where young women and girls tend to have little say when it comes to condom use.

Information and discussion of sexual and reproductive health as well as contraception itself were largely inaccessible. None of the young participants in this study had discussed sex or contraception with their parents or older family members. School sex education was not mentioned by any of the participants. Some of the young participants were aware of contraception and where they may be able to access it, but said that fear of lack of confidentiality was the biggest barrier. As Cara stated:

> I didn't think of using that [condoms] because I was scared in case I might go to the hospital and ask for it and the nurses will ask me why I'm asking for it.
>
> (Cara, pregnant at 17, Tongatapu)

Heather was also deterred from accessing condoms from a non-government organisation, as her cousin worked there:

> It's hard, because I know this is the only place where we could get them for free. But since she is my cousin, I couldn't … She might tell my mum.
>
> (Heather, pregnant at 18, Vava'u)

Most participants were reluctant to access contraception. Reluctance was accentuated and compounded by societal expectations that young women should not inquire or seek this sort of information. In general, young people do not have access to reliable and accurate information on sexual and reproductive health and contraception. The subject is rarely discussed at home. The only information available to most of the interviewees was from the Internet, and in particular through social media. Lack of knowledge about reproductive health and inaccessibility to contraception contributed to unplanned pregnancies.

### *Reactions to unplanned pregnancies: surprise, fear and denial*

The first physical symptoms of pregnancy came as a surprise to all of the young women and girls and they described being frightened and not knowing what to do when they realised that they were pregnant. Because they were scared, most did not confirm their pregnancy or have any interaction with a health service until they were four or five months pregnant, sometimes even later. Reactions to unplanned pregnancy are described in the accounts of these young women and girls.

Brooke suspected that she was pregnant when she started to experience symptoms, but she did not tell anyone. When questioned by her mother, she lied:

> … I didn't know that I was pregnant. I kind of have a feeling that I was because the food and my lunch, I used to eat them and it's not like before. I see there's changes and difference. When I have my lunch with my friends they would eat, and I don't like that food anymore. I kept touching my stomach and I wonder if I'm pregnant when I have this feeling like morning sickness and those things … my mum told me, 'You never told me you needed some pads. You haven't got your period or anything?' Then I said umm no, no. It's just something. I'm not pregnant.
>
> (Brooke, pregnant at 18, Tongatapu)

Fran's aunty helped her have a pregnancy test and confirm her pregnancy after Fran noticed her tummy growing. Fran did not want to tell her parents:

> Probably around October I started not having my period, but I didn't even think I was pregnant. I thought it was just nothing. I started vomiting. I started having those pregnant symptoms and then maybe around January my tummy started to grow and then I went to get a pregnancy test and, yes, it was positive. That's the time I knew I was pregnant.
>
> (Fran, pregnant at 17, Tongatapu)

Georgia's grandmother took her to the hospital for a pregnancy test. Georgia recounts her feelings when the doctor confirmed that she was pregnant and asked to speak with her parents:

> I was crying that day.'Cause it's all my fault, I didn't tell it to my parents. And the first moment that the doctor told me that he wants to talk with my parents. That's the first time I can't hold my tears, when I heard that the doctor is going to be telling my parents that I'm pregnant.
>
> (Georgia, pregnant at 18, Vava'u)

Many participants continued to lie to their mother and father even after they found out that they were pregnant.

> … it gets to a time my skirt didn't fit anymore over my belly and my mother asked if something is wrong and I told her no … my mother asked me if I already have my period and I said no because she is the one who does the washing. Then she told me we should go with my father to the hospital and have a check-up, and the doctor told me to come in alone for my examination, so my father waited outside. I found out I'm pregnant and came to my father and told him something else. I lied to him because I was scared.
>
> (Debra, pregnant at 17, Tongatapu)

### *Family and community attitudes towards the pregnancy*

All participants said they were scared to tell their parents they were pregnant, and most initially lied when questioned by their parents about possible pregnancy. However, the narratives of the young women show that although families are disappointed and often initially angry, immediate family members and close relatives usually comprise the key support throughout pregnancy and beyond. Aunties, female cousins and grandmothers are the first people to be confided in or informed about an unplanned pregnancy. Older women in the study pointed out that:

> *Ko e 'uluaki 'api ako ko 'api* (home is the first school) *pea ko e 'uluaki faiako 'a e matu'a* (parents are the first teachers).

Tongans perceive that it is the parents' role to teach their children, but young women are not being taught about sexual and reproductive health by their parents, or by other family members.

In most situations, the parents' initial reaction was anger, disappointment and hurt. Several participants expressed that their fear was even greater because their parents were figureheads in their church. However, in most cases, the parents' anger and disappointment changed to love and support.

Kelly was scared because of what her father would do if he found out she was pregnant, and then when he did he pressured her to terminate the pregnancy:

> I was so scared of what would happen if my dad found out … When he found out he was trying to tell me to abort the baby. He forced me to take medicine, he forced me to drink strong tea and strong coffee … When I woke up one morning, he had made it, he told me to just take the cup and come to his room, and he told me to sit down beside him and drink all of it. It tasted like … strong … different … I drank the tea, and he also told me don't eat any food from the morning'til evening … he just gave me Panadol, five to six Panadol to take … maybe two times a day. However, I only took the medicine one time, and when he told me to take it the second time, I rushed to my room and threw it away … It's not only my father who told me to abort the baby. Even my aunty … she was angry at me, she also told me to abort the baby. When he gave me all those things and forced me to take it, I thought, is he a good father or not? Sometimes I thought, how would he feel if this was his child? Did he ever do this to his wife when she was pregnant? That's what I was thinking [participant crying].
>
> (Kelly, pregnant at 18, Vava'u)

The young women and girls' fear had more to do with the social stigma and disrepute the pregnancy brought to their parents and their family's social standing in their community. The fear was deeper if their parents were heavily involved in the church.

Out of fear of being judged, one participant's father explicitly told her not to 'get rid' of the unborn baby because of his role in the church.

> My mum comforted me, and I apologised to her about the lies. She said it's okay, it's just she's annoyed about me lying to her … At times, I do regret not being obedient to my parents because of what has transpired, so I try my best now to be obedient … When my father found out, he was angry. He sat me down and he asked me all these questions about what happened to me. He said that I should have made better choices because of his role at church. The people at our church will point a finger at him not being a better parent and it sort of embarrassed him. But then he encouraged me to be brave and not to try to get rid of the baby because they will provide everything for my baby, and it will be their first grandchild.
>
> (Angela, pregnant at 16, Tongatapu)

Angela's story shows that in many cases concern about community opinion outweighs the needs of the family, speaking to the social significance of the hierarchical structure of Tongan society.

While Tongan families tend to be strict in raising their children and expect that their daughters will not have an unplanned pregnancy, most families, in this study, did come around to support and care for their daughters or granddaughters.

> I have my grandmother, sister and my cousins, my big sister. Yeah. Them. They taught me how to become a mum ... I just have that feeling that my child gave me more strength and it made me not give up life. It's one thing that I'm living for and that's why I love becoming a mum. When I had my child, I feel like he gave my life more meaning, how to live life, why I'm still living.
>
> (Fran, pregnant at 17, Tongatapu)

A lot of the young women and girls described that when they gave birth and saw their baby, they had an overwhelming sense of purpose, meaning and love in their life as a mother. And although many of the young women and girls described initially experiencing disappointment and anger from their parents, once born the baby was commonly valued and loved in the family, and the young women and girls were provided with financial and emotional support in their role as a new mother.

## Discussion: talanoa (discussion) of the taboo?

The study data reconfirm that discussion of sexual and reproductive health is taboo in most family and community contexts in Tonga, and that accurate, reliable and locally specific information is neither easily accessible nor readily shared with young people, not even at schools (see also Ali-Traill, Chapter 2; Veukiso-Ulugia et al., Chapter 3; Futter-Puati, Chapter 4). Consequently, they have low knowledge and limited access to confidential sexual and reproductive health information and services including contraception. Condoms were the only contraceptive method that most of the young women and girls interviewed were aware of prior to their pregnancy. Moreover, the young women and girls seldom initiated or controlled the use of this method — which was typically the prerogative of their male partner.

Christian religious beliefs, traditional values, taboos and gender expectations limit young women and girls' agency within their relationships, and lead to societal vulnerability by constraining their ability to make informed sexual and reproductive decisions. The young women and girls' narratives demonstrate how, similar to other Pacific and international contexts, male partners tend to have more control over the terms of their relationships, including decision-making about condom use. Age-related expectations about premarital sex and gender norms as social influences play a role in deterring young women from accessing and using contraception. Age and gender expectations also shape their reactions and their families' reactions to unplanned pregnancy. Lack of feminine agency around condom use and low knowledge of other contraceptive options increases individual risk of unintentionally becoming pregnant. Once pregnant, barriers to communicating with family members exacerbate isolation and fear for young women and delay access to their most significant support system.

We propose talanoa as a means of potentially reducing the individual risk of unplanned pregnancy through the sharing of knowledge and also as a way of addressing societal vulnerability through discussing gender social norms. Talanoa, the Tongan word for talking, dialogue or having a conversation, could be used as a means to facilitate intergenerational discussion on sexual and reproductive health. *Fofola e fala ka e talanoa e kāinga* (roll out the mat so that the family can talk), is a Tongan metaphor where family members are invited to gather and talk (Tuinukuafe et al. 2012; Lino 2015). Talanoa is ideally inclusive and interactive and can foster increased understanding. It signifies, '*Ta e lango kei mama'o,*' (better to be prepared ahead of time) (Havea et al. 2019), which in Tongan embodies the importance of prevention or resilience in anticipation of an issue or problem.

A recent evaluation of a family violence intervention and prevention programme targeting the Tongan community in Aotearoa New Zealand, documented the use of *fofola e fala ka e talanoa e kāinga* (roll out the mat so that the family can engage in a discussion or dialogue), as a Pacific-indigenous approach to support efforts to curtail violence within families (Havea et al. 2021). Havea et al. (2021) evoke the mat as a refuge and safe place for people to express their feelings:

> the mat offers an intentional cultural enclave within which Tongan social hierarchical relations are suspended, though not totally absent, for a time ... the enactment of hierarchical social structure is discouraged so that every person has an opportunity to voice their concerns and to be heard - this includes children.
>
> (Havea et al. 2021, p. 5)

Just as the mat has been utilised as a space for discussion of the sensitive issue of family violence it may also enable discussion of sexual and reproductive health.

A key recommendation in the Tonga Adolescent Unplanned Pregnancy study is for sexual and reproductive health and contraceptive education to be delivered to both older women and young women and girls together, and in a forum that enables the older women to take some ownership of the process. Talanoa on relationships, contraception and gender roles could be facilitated between older and younger women. This may push the boundaries of what is culturally acceptable, but could also allow young women and girls to have a voice, discuss gender social norms and learn about taboo subjects such as sex and contraceptives through intergenerational discussion. This could include hosting of small mother-and-daughter group meetings or workshops aiming to improve and begin to normalise dialogue between mothers and their daughters on matters of gender, sexuality, sexual relationships and reproductive decision-making and health. Discussion of topics such as sexuality and sexual relationships are forbidden in mixed-sex company; having separate female and male talanoa would be more socially acceptable (Guttenbeil-Likiliki 2006). Talanoa among older men and young men and boys may also provide an opportunity for sharing of knowledge and discussion about sexual and reproductive health and gender relations among males.

## Conclusion

Traditional social and cultural expectations of young women and girls' sexual behaviour and relationships conflict with social media and other global youth culture messages. The participants' narratives of unplanned pregnancy and sexual and reproductive health show various areas where Tongan cultural norms hinder discussion, within the family, of sexual relationships and reproductive health. Young women tend to rely instead on the, sometimes dubious, information they can access in privacy, pointing to the need for accurate and culturaly relevant information, even on social media (see Ali-Traill, Chapter 2).

Increased access to information and condoms alone may have limited benefit in reducing unplanned pregnancy among young women and girls unless gendered power dynamics are also addressed in a manner that furthers the confidence and ability of young women to effectively negotiate condom use with sexual partners. Constraints on female voice extend well beyond the family mat; the 2021 elections in Tonga saw the formation of a government with not a single woman included. Ensuring that women, young women and girls in particular, have not just a 'place' on the mat but also a 'voice' will be a challenge in Tonga; a challenge to government and civil society institutions and to public and private practices. Talanoa may provide a culturally appropriate means to facilitate intergenerational discussion on sexual and reproductive health and relationship issues of concern to young women in Tonga; a place to not only share information but also to consider gender roles and expectations in a way that is inclusive of the experiences and voices of Tongan young women and girls.

## Notes

1 Not her real name. All participant names have been changed. Names have been anglicised to reduce the chance of a quotation being attributed to another young woman in Tonga.

2 The Tongan word for talking, dialogue or having a conversation. Talanoa is ideally inclusive and interactive and can foster increased understanding.

3 The three-country study — *Adolescent unplanned pregnancy in the Pacific* — was commissioned by Pacific Women Shaping Pacific Development, an aid programme funded by the Government of Australia's Department of Foreign Affairs and Trade. Permission was granted by Pacific Women Shaping Pacific Development to use the data from the Tongan study for this chapter. We extend our appreciation to Pacific Women and Vanesa Heleta of Talitha Project, Tonga for their support for this project including feedback on this chapter and encouragement to disseminate findings in this way.

## References


Austin, L., 2013. *Talanoa radio: exploring the interface of development, culture and community radio in the South Pacific*. PhD thesis. The University of Queensland. Available from: https://www.academia.edu/39670286/Talanoa_Radio_Exploring_the_Interface_of_Development_Culture_and_Community_Radio_in_the_South_Pacific [Accessed 17 January 2022].

Bell, S. and Aggleton, P., 2013. Social influences on young people's sexual health in Uganda. *Health Education*, 113 (2), 102–114. doi:10.1108/09654281311298795

Bell, S., et al., 2018. Youth-centred research to help prevent and mitigate the adverse health and social impacts of pregnancy amongst young Papua New Guineans. *Reproductive Health Matters*, 26 (54), 5–12. doi:10.1080/09688080.2018.1512297

Butt, L. and Munro, J. 2007. Rebel girls? Unplanned pregnancy and colonialism in highlands Papua, Indonesia. *Culture, Health & Sexuality*, 9 (6), 585–598. doi:1080/13691050701515324

Futter-Puati, D.M., 2017. *Api'ianga tupuanga kopapa: Sexuality education in the Cook Islands*. PhD thesis. RMIT University. Available from: https://researchrepository.rmit.edu.au/esploro/outputs/doctoral/Apiianga-tupuanga-kopapa-sexuality-education-in-the-Cook-Islands/9921863878301341 [Accessed 17 January 2022]

Guttenbeil-Likiliki, O., 2006. Advancing women's representation in Tonga: Research to advance women's political representation in Forum island countries. In: E. Huffer (ed), *A woman's place is in the House – the House of Parliament*. Suva, Fiji: Pacific Islands Forum Secretariat, 144–208.

Havea, P., et al., 2019. Tā e Lango' kei Mama'o: A framework for resilience development in Tonga. *SSRN Electronic Journal*. doi:10.2139/ssrn.3403372

Havea, S., Alefaio-Tugia, S., and Hodgetts, D., 2021. *Fofola e Fala ka e Talanoa Kainga:* A Tongan approach to family violence prevention and intervention. *Journal of Pacific Rim Psychology*, 15, 1–12. doi:10.1177/18344909211040866

Kelly, A., et al., 2010. Gendered talk about sex, sexual relationships and HIV among young people in Papua New Guinea. *Culture, Health & Sexuality*, 12 (3), 221–232. doi:10.1080/13691050903181107

Kennedy, E., et al., 2014. 'These issues aren't talked about at home': A qualitative study of the sexual and reproductive health information preferences of adolescents in Vanuatu. *BMC Public Health*, 14 (770). doi:10.1186/1471-2458-14-770

Linhart, C., et al., 2020. Adolescent unplanned pregnancy in the Pacific: Tonga. Sydney: School of Public Health and Community Medicine, UNSW. Available from: http://unsworks.unsw.edu.au/fapi/datastream/unsworks:73177/bin48387be0-8558-48dc-8257-552c1237c3b0?view=true&xy=01 [Accessed 17 January 2022].

Lino, A., 2015. *Fofola e fala kae alea e kāinga: Exploring the issues of communication regarding Tongan youth suicide in South Auckland, New Zealand 'Aulola he-polealisi fuka lino*. MA thesis. Auckland University of Technology.

McMillan, K., Linhart, C., Gorman, H., Kepa, B., et al., 2020. Adolescent unplanned pregnancy in the Pacific: Vanuatu. Sydney: School of Public Health and Community Medicine, UNSW. Available from: http://unsworks.unsw.edu.au/fapi/datastream/unsworks:73998/bin504dac16-9ed4–4186-a28b-932f5c50e6b0?view=true&xy=01 [Accessed 17 Jan 2022].

McMillan, K., Linhart, C., Gorman, H., Kim, M., et al., 2020. Adolescent unplanned pregnancy in the Pacific: Chuuk. Sydney: School of Public Health and Community Medicine, UNSW. Available from: http://unsworks.unsw.edu.au/fapi/datastream/unsworks:73685/bin7a4299a5–9b2f-42a9-8eac-58e42d5ed94b?view=true&xy=01 [Accessed 17 Jan 2022].

McMillan, K.E., 2011. Tradition, respect and reputation: cultural, familial, and personal risk attached to condom use for young people in Tonga. *Intersections: Gender and Sexuality in Asia and the Pacific*, 26, (August). http://intersections.anu.edu.au/issue26/mcmillan.htm

McMillan, K. and Worth, H., 2011. The impact of socio-cultural context on young people's condom use: Evidence from two Pacific Island countries. *Culture, Health & Sexuality*, 13 (3), 313–326. doi:10.1080/13691058.2010.529945

Mitchell, E. and Bennett, L.R., 2020. Young women's perceptions and experiences of sexual risk in Suva, Fiji. *Culture, Health & Sexuality*, 22 (5), 504–519. doi:10.1080/13691058.2019.1614669

O'Connor, M. 2018. *Tiko Bulabula: Understanding and measuring adolescent sexual and reproductive well-being in Fiji Islands*. PhD thesis. UNSW Sydney. doi:10.26190/unsworks/20901

O'Connor, M., et al., 2018. Understanding the meaning of youth sexual and reproductive well-being in Fiji. *Culture, Health & Sexuality*, 20 (11), 1244–1258. doi: 10.1080/13691058.2018.1424938

Reed, S.J., et al., 2017. Honoring motherhood: The meaning of childbirth for Tongan women. *The American Journal of Maternal/Child Nursing*, 42 (3), 146–152. doi:10.1097/NMC.0000000000000328

Sorchik R., et al., 2019. *Fertility trends in Pacific Island countries and territories*. Noumea: Secretariat of the Pacific Community. Available from: https://sdd.spc.int/news/2019/07/19/fertility-trends-pacific-island-countries-and-territories [Accessed 17 January 2022].

Tonga Statistics Department, 2020. *Tonga multiple indicator cluster survey 2019, survey findings report*. Nuku'alofa, Tonga: Tonga Statistics Department. Available from: https://tongastats.gov.to/survey/mics-survey/ [Accessed 17 January 2022].

Tonga Statistics Department, 2021. Tonga Statistics Department [online]. Available from: https://tongastats.gov.to/ [Accessed 15 December 2021].

Tuinukuafe, T., et al., 2012. *Fofola e fala kae talanoa e kainga: A Tongan conceptual framework for the prevention of and intervention in family violence in New Zealand – Famili Lelei*. In: Nga vaka o kāiga tapu: A Pacific conceptual framework to address family violence in New Zealand. Available from: https://www.pasefikaproud.co.nz/assets/Resources-for-download/PasefikaProudResource-Nga-Vaka-o-Kaiga-Tapu-Main-Pacific-Framework.pdf [Accessed 22 April 2022].

UNESCO, 2022. *Tonga education and literacy* [online]. UNESCO Institute of Statistics. Available from: http://uis.unesco.org/en/country/to [Accessed 29 January 2022].

United Nations Population Fund (UNFPA), 2013. *Moana Declaration: outcome statement of Pacific parliamentarians for population & development*. Suva, Fiji: UNFPA. Available from: https://pacific.unfpa.org/sites/default/files/resource-pdf/PACIFICCONFERENCEOFPARLIAMENTARIANSFORADVOCACYONICPDBEYOND2014OutcomeStatement.pdf [Accessed 10 January 2022].

United Nations Population Fund (UNFPA), 2015. *Kingdom of Tonga sexual and reproductive health rights needs assessment*. April 2015. Suva, Fiji: UNFPA. Available from: https://pacific.unfpa.org/sites/default/files/pub-pdf/1.KingdomofTongaSexualandReproductiveHealthRights-NeedsAssessmentReportLRv1.pdf [Accessed 10 January 2022].

Vaioleti T.M., 2006. Talanoa research methodology: a developing position on Pacific research. *Waikato Journal of Education*, 12, 21–34. doi:10.15663/wje.v12i1.296

White, A.L., Mann, E.S., and Larkan, F., 2018a. Contraceptive knowledge, attitudes, and use among adolescent mothers in the Cook Islands. *Sexual & Reproductive Healthcare*, 16, 92–97.

White, A.L., Mann, E.S., and Larkan, F., 2018b. 'You just have to learn to keep moving on': Young women's experiences with unplanned pregnancy in the Cook Islands. *Culture, Health & Sexuality*, 20 (7), 731–745. doi:10.1080/13691058.2017.1371336

Part III

# Belonging, connectedness and justice

# 11 Moana masculinities in the diaspora: Cultural identity and performance on the dance stage and the sports field

*Roannie Ng Shiu, Asetoa Sam Pilisi and David Taufui Mikato Fa'avae*

*O ai le Toa, o ai le Toa? Samoa!*
Who are the Warriors, who are the Warriors? Samoa!

*Tuia tuia tuia, I'm a Keke Boy.*
Stab, stab, stab, I'm a Keke Boy

## Introduction

Pacific men and their bodies have long fascinated Others. Through settler-colonialism and the arrival of European visitors and settlers, the writers and observers have viewed Pacific men as 'adorned bodies' rather than social and intellectual beings who possess critical and intellectual subjectivities beyond the deficit native narratives often portrayed by those outside of Indigenous *moana* ocean localities (Hokowhitu 2004; Jolly 2008; Tengan 2008). Our Pacific men are noble savages and warriors and conceptualisations of moana masculinities highlight the nuanced ways in which power, place and performance are shaped within diasporic Pacific communities today. The deficit tropes developed by Europeans in the nineteenth century continue today, across our vast moana, with Pacific men often being viewed as deeply physical, natural sportsmen, but academically inept (Hokowhitu 2004). This dominant discourse serves to 'limit, homogenize and reproduce an acceptable and imagined' (Hokowhitu, 2004, p. 262) Pacific masculinity of a particular type. As a result of colonisation, mobility and migration, many Pacific men are now born and raised away from their ancestral lands in the moana. This disconnect presents challenges for many Pacific men including the preservation and celebration of culture and language in new lands together with limiting hegemonic discourses about what it means to be a 'man from the moana' as part of the diaspora.[1]

Migration across the moana has a long, sometimes troubled, history with indentured labour from the Pacific to Australia playing a significant role. It has been estimated that between 1863 and 1906 (Halter 2015) almost 61,000 indentured labourers from the Pacific Islands were taken to work in Queensland on sugar cane plantations. Most came from New Caledonia, Vanuatu and the

DOI: 10.4324/9781003142072-14

Solomon Islands, as well as from the Torres Strait Islands and were forced to work in slavery through a process referred to as 'blackbirding' (Halter 2015). The descendants of the Pacific trade labourers in Queensland are often referred to as South Sea Islanders and include prominent rugby league figures such as Mal Meninga and Wendell Sailor. Elsewhere in the Pacific, patterns of migration typically align with the colonial past. For example, migration to the USA has largely been from Micronesia and American Samoa. In Aotearoa-NZ, the largest migrant groups come from Samoa and Tonga and the Pacific states with free association (Niue, Tokelau and the Cook Islands).

After the Second World War, Aotearoa-NZ encouraged the mass migration of Pacific islanders into the country, to help address labour shortages in a growing economy. The influx of Pacific islanders from the 1950s to the mid-1970s meant Aotearoa-NZ was able to meet the much-needed demand for skilled and semi-skilled workers, particularly in the manufacturing sector and in building Aotearoa-NZ's infrastructure (Spoonley and Bedford 2012). Mass migration was enabled by chain migration whereby, after one or two Pacific households had established themselves new country with secure housing and employment, additional family members from the Pacific would then migrate (Macpherson 2004).

Despite Australia's colonial legacy in the Western Pacific, particularly in Papua New Guinea, migration from the Pacific to Australia has been limited in comparison to Aotearoa-NZ and the USA (Pryke 2014). This can be explained by Australia's 'White Australia' policy between 1901 to 1973 which intentionally restricted non-European immigration. It was also due to the fact that Australia did not have free-association with former colonies in the way Aotearoa-NZ does. In more recent history, the Trans-Tasman Travel Arrangement, introduced in 1973, has facilitated the migration to Australia of a significant number of Pacific Islanders with Aotearoa-NZ citizenship.

Irrespective of whether they were migrants from their place of cultural heritage, or were born in a third country before migration, people of Pacific heritage have established important communities in the diaspora. The main motivation for this migration has been to seek economic, employment and educational opportunities (Ng Shiu 2011). However, recent examination of the experiences of Pacific transnational communities has revealed that the idea of migration leading to better socioeconomic position has in most cases been a fantasy rather than a reality. Pacific transnational communities in urban cities experience significant educational, health and social inequalities and inequities. Added to this has been the loss of language, ongoing challenges with cultural identity (Macpherson 2004; Ng Shiu 2011), and a sense of loneliness that comes from being away from home.

Engagement in competitive sport and traditional dance is intimately related to these patterns of migration, with Pacific men developing particular interests depending on where they live, as well as their colonial history (Panapa and Phillips 2014; Uperesa 2014). In this chapter we examine these involvements and their implications for ideas and practices of masculinity among modern moana men in the diaspora through a focus on Pacific warrior performers and Pacific male athletes. We present two case studies, the first of the Niue *Takalo* (warrior dance) performance at Polyfest,[2] and the second, Pacific male rugby league athletes in in the diaspora. In these case studies we examine efforts to reframe the 'Pacific warrior' through cultural empowerment paradigms for men living away from their ancestral lands. By examining contemporary gender ideals for and of Pacific men, we seek to decolonise and disrupt the discourses that reinforce the view that our men are noble savages and warriors and provide a more nuanced understanding of power, place and performance in shaping moana masculinities today.

## Men (and masculinity) of the moana – theoretical framework

Moana masculinities emerge in relation to and sometimes in resistance to the hegemonic forces of colonialism, imperialism and militarism (Hokowhitu 2014; Tengan 2008). The powerful expression of masculinities in the moana connects embodied memories with gendered places and the sexualised flow of time (Jolly 2008). Bodies are a discursive text on which ethnicity, sexuality and gender are inscribed. Gender is socially ascribed and socially produced, often in binary ways, masculine or feminine. As culturally produced binary expressions of gender, Pacific brown male bodies are constructed within a deeply complex set of socio-cultural and socio-political meanings and practices. However, as Indigenous scholars of masculinity argue, dominant ideas of gender, masculinity and femininity tend to be monocultural and Eurocentric, far removed from the lived experiences of Indigenous communities (Hokowhitu 2014; Fa'avae et al. 2021). Tengan (2002), for example, argues Indigenous masculinities require a process of decolonisation through the restructuring of gender meanings and practices, informed by Indigenous philosophies.

Using the concepts of *vā*,[3] which refers to social connections and relationships as well as relational space, or space in-between (see Wendt 1996), and the Niuean concept of *vahaloto* which refers to 'time and place, as well as the space between and among people' (Vilitama 2015, p. 258), both of which constitute the critical spaces in which ethical relational becoming occurs, the sense-making of power and performance for Pacific men can be understood as a grounded practice that requires negotiation and navigation (Fa'avae et al. 2021). Hokowhitu (2016) has used Indigenous studies to critically examine the ways in which Indigenous masculinities and other Indigeno-centric practices are presented as having a fixed meaning or authenticity, claiming,

> we need to understand our embodiment as manifestations of knowledge insurrections, to make a new story of unintelligibility and of radical intent, refusing the Western demand to be an all-knowing subject that believes it masters what it knows.
>
> (cited in Moreton-Robinson 2016, p. 13)

There exists a paucity of literature on men and masculinity from across the moana. Most current literature focuses on Papua New Guinea (see for example,

Sai 2007; Gibbs 2016) and Indigenous men in Hawai'i (see for example, Tengan 2002, 2016; Young 2017) and Aotearoa-NZ (see for example, Hokowhitu 2004, 2014; Hamley and Grice 2021). In consequence, there is a lack of literature on what healthy masculinity might mean from an Indigenous moana perspective. The challenge for developing a Pacific or moana Indigenous framework lies partly in terminology and partly in the different cultures the moana men feel connected to, and to which they can relate. The use of Pasifika as a pan-ethnic identity to describe various Pacific communities in Aotearoa-NZ (and increasingly in Australia) was intended to offer a more inclusive descriptor of those who subscribed to the Pacific Way (Anae 1997). The irony, however, is that many communities from the Western Pacific do not relate to or identify with the term Pasifika, highlighting the problems in trying to create a pan-ethnic identity. Trying to understand what it means to be a Pacific or Moana man is therefore both complex and contextual. We attempt to engage with some of this complexity and contextuality in what follows. We begin by focusing on cultural empowerment through dance, exploring Takalo and Polyfest as cultural sites in which performance and language hold significance. We then examine cultural empowerment through sport, particularly within the context of rugby league football and framings of masculinities.

## Takalo and Polyfest – what it means to be a man

The *Takalo* is a traditional Niue pre-war dance and challenge. Contemporary performances of this cultural practice can be problematic as the dance is often linked to Captain James Cook's racist portrayal of Niue men as 'savages.' In 1774, when Cook tried to land in Niue he was met by a group of men who were wary of outsiders (Talagi 1982). Cook is said to have misinterpreted the pre-war challenge by the men which was in the form of a dance, posed as one of outright aggression, which led to Cook labelling the island he had reached as the Savage Island (Talagi 1982). In contrast, other cultures that Cook and other colonisers visited were different, with Tonga, for example, being declared by Cook as the Friendly Isles. The damage created by this negative colonial framing of men lingers on within Niue communities, leaving little room to advance more welcoming and peaceful forms of masculinity, especially among those born and living abroad. These historical descriptions and their legacy serve as reminders of the power colonial empires have to name and shame Pacific men and women. Today, early career Niuean scholars are actively working to shift the power relations at play here and ensure that Pacific Islanders in general, and Pacific men in particular, have the opportunity to name themselves (Pilisi 2020; Aleke-Fa'avae et al. 2021).

For young Pacific performers, there is no bigger stage on which to showcase the power and elegance of Pacific dance than Polyfest. Polyfest is a performing arts festival that is the largest of its kind in the world and cultural dance is a key component of it. It started in 1974 as a secondary school event for students in Auckland, Aotearoa-NZ with just four schools participating. Today the festival includes over 9,000 performers and attracts over 100,000 spectators. Utilising the concepts of vā (Wendt 1996) and vahaloto (Vilitama 2015) to examine Polyfest and its impact on Aotearoa-NZ born Pacific youth, it is possible to understand the event as one in which concepts of gender, power and masculinity are negotiated. While there is already an important body of literature examining the place of cultural identity within the festival (see for example, Mackley-Crump 2015; Anayo 2017; Williams 2018), nothing to date has focused on Pacific masculinity and the power of performance. On the different stages at Polyfest (Samoan, Tongan, Cook Islands and Niuean) we can see male bodies adorned, painted and clothed in traditional attire as storytelling unfolds in new and different ways.

Performing on the stage at Polyfest is a highlight of the year for Niue youth. It is one of the few opportunities Niue youth in Aotearoa-NZ get to be surrounded by Niue culture and language (Togiatama-Otto 2019). For anyone who has visited the Niue Polyfest stage or seen the performance, the dominant depiction of Niue masculinity in most performances remains one of staged aggression. Because the festival provides the biggest platform of its kind for Niue people and for men to dance, this portrayal is amplified so as to constitute the essentialist trope of the Niue man. Young men find themselves caught up in reinforcing this colonial imagery. Away from Polyfest and across our dynamic Niue communities, particularly among Niue youth, we see how savage imagery has offered as a unique identifier and a source of pride on clothing, social media posts, rap lyrics and the sports arena (Aleke-Fa'avae et al. 2021).

### *Working with masculinities – cultural empowerment for men through performance and language?*

Beyond Polyfest, there are limited opportunities for Aotearoa-NZ born Niue men to engage with Niue language and culture (Tagata Pasifika 2020) to develop other forms of masculinity. Given that Niue language use has been declining in the Aotearoa-NZ Niue community and features on the UNESCO endangered languages list (Moseley 2010), the current cultural landscape for Niue people in Aotearoa-NZ is a challenging one to navigate.

The relational concepts of vā and vahaloto enable an appreciation of how Niue men relate to historical and contemporary accounts of what being a man is about. Cook's interpretation of Niue masculinity left a lasting impression, with aggression (staged and otherwise) remaining a marker of Niue masculinity today. Despite the paucity of writing on Niue masculinity, the existing literature paints a picture in which heavy alcohol consumption is seen as a marker of manhood (Nosa et al. 2011). The connection between Niue masculinity and alcohol misuse can be seen in Niue rapper Diggy Dupe's Keke Boy lyrics, 'Tama Niue, inu hake, Son of Niue, drink up/have a drink' (Atutolu 2020). Togiatama-Otto (2019) highlights the significance of *tutala* (discussion, conversation) as a cultural practice that help Niue male secondary school students understand their experiences within schooling, and the place of cultural identity and *magafaoa* (family) in career aspirations. Unpacking Niue masculinity using Niue approaches and concepts like vahaloto as relational space, enable close articulations of the Niue person and its nuanced interpretation across the diaspora.

Back home in Niue, and more strongly connected to the *fonua* (land) and moana, Niue men immerse themselves in vā connections within the vahaloto space of relating. This is evident through their connections across relational spaces linked to friendships, family and community, having a wider set of opportunities to develop and express themselves as Niue men. Both traditional and contemporary practices on the island include fishing in hand-made timber canoes, tending to family gardens and plantations of staple foods such as taro and coconut, and learning and fulfilling leadership roles within their families, villages and church communities. As is common in village life, young Niue men observe their fathers and other older men in learning to be a man and assuming their gendered responsibilities. In contrast, for men living in urban Aotearoa-NZ the cultural landscape is not the same, so access to socio-cultural activities and resources grounded in Niue fonua are challenging in the diaspora. Polyfest and Takalo are among the few activities that share Niue knowledge and practices relevant to understanding Niue masculinity on Aotearoa-NZ land.

To address the unmet needs of Niue men in Aotearoa-NZ's diaspora in relation to gender, identity and health, Aleke-Fa'avae et al. (2021) work with the Ponataki e Atu Toa Niue project to seek to identify and create alternative ways of connecting with cultural identity and masculinity. The project aims to be solution-focused and part of this work uses the traditional Takalo war dance as a cultural tool for empowerment and cultural reconnection. Utilising digital vā (Muliaumaseali'i 2017) to create an online space in which Niue men can learn about the project and connect through shared cultural experiences, a Facebook group has been developed. In the first week of the group going live, more than 500 Niue men joined, confirming both the value of using digital vā in linking men together across places and spaces. To add cultural legitimacy to the project, Aleke-Fa'avae et al. (2021) sought out the expertise of a well-known *asafo* (artistic composer), Lavea Puheke, who resides in Niue, to compose a Takalo that would bridge the cultural divide between tagata Niue at home and abroad in the diaspora. A staged performance of the Takalo is available on YouTube (see https://www.youtube.com/watch?v=1nqxMWE2OGk).

Through the work of the project and building on the terminology used by Fehoko (2016) workers sought to create a 'cultural classroom' for Niue men. We encouraged the use of *vagahau Niue* (Niue language) and other cultural customs that would normally take place in the village or church. Often during the introductions or debrief sessions, many men would apologise for their lack of vagahau Niue skills. In responding to these ongoing apologies, we adopted a 'come as you are approach' to ensure that whatever competency in the Niue language or culture men had, all were welcomed in the classroom and considered 'Niuean enough.' This contributed to creating a culturally safe space in which Aotearoa-NZ born Niue young men's lived experiences were acknowledged rather than diminished, and a strengths-based approach to learning was encouraged.

The normalising of Niue language use and re-enactment of cultural customs, be this digitally or in person, are powerful wins in contributing to evolving narratives of Niue masculinity. Cultural experiences that uplift rather than shame Aotearoa-NZ born Niue men encourage connection to heritage, language and customs and, most importantly, to oneself when the question '*Ko hai au?*' (Who am I?) is asked. Ultimately, what became clear from this project was that by working together men can create culturally affirming spaces – by Niue men, for Niue men. Truthfully, only Aotearoa-NZ born Niue men can speak to lived experiences away from Niue and the yearning and wanting to belong they experience despite cultural challenges inherited from earlier generations. When given the licence to speak out and document these narratives through dance and in other ways, this journey empowers Niue men to be confident in their own stories and be ready to share them with brothers, sons and generations to come.

## Masculine intersections at play – on and off the field

We turn now to a rather different but related context – namely Pacific men's engagement with sport in Australia. Pacific communities make up less than one percent of the total population in Australia yet their members are significantly represented in sports such Rugby League at both junior and professional levels. Recent estimates suggest that fully 46% of all players in Junior Rugby League in Australia are of Pacific Islander heritage (One Wellbeing 2021). At the same time, players' agents and coaches actively seek Pacific talent encouraging young Pacific men still in their mid-teens to join the diaspora for the opportunity to secure a contract. Often relocation takes the form of migration from Aotearoa-NZ to Australia. For young Pacific men, the pressure of trying to 'make it,' compounded by living away from home with limited family connections and social ties, carries significant implications for their health and well-being, triggering mental health problems and even suicide (Cadzow 2013). While Pacific Islanders play an important role within the sport as players, it is largely white men who have power over the game through their roles as club owners, coaches and senior management. This unequal relationship between the players at the centre of the sport and these power holders influences Pacific men's displays of masculinity on the field.

The hypervisibility of Pacific men is perhaps most evident in the pre-game rituals, epitomised by the *haka* war dance that precedes rugby union or rugby league fixtures involving teams from the moana such as the Aotearoa-NZ All Blacks. The pre-game haka has become a modern-day ritual preparing 'warriors' for the sports battlefield. The Aotearoa-NZ All Blacks are believed to have first performed a syncretised haka called the Ka Mate in 1888–89 during international tours to the UK and Australia (All Blacks Experience 2022) and the haka continues to be performed to global audiences today. In the same way that the All Blacks incorporated traditional history into modern day performances of the haka, so too do other teams from the moana including the Tongan Rugby Team with the Sipi Tau, the Samoan team with the Siva Tau, and the Fijian Rugby team with the Cibi. These pre-game rituals are not new, but rather evolving sites of performance and expression of Pacific masculinity, with non-Pacific Islanders in these teams learning how to perform them.

Pre-game haka rituals present physical assertions of strength and power through voice projection and bodily movements choreographed to demonstrate warriors' intent to assuage their team's appetite for a triumphant battle. The pre-game haka is a highly emotive exchange of challenges to encourage opponents and onlookers to feel intimidated and excited for the battle ahead. The scripted war cries set the scene for the dramatic theatre that will unfold in an unpredictable contest between warring parties. Nowadays, professional sports fixtures are broadcast to a global audience but in consequence Pacific men become constrained by this portrayal, with the pre-game haka exchanges and the ensuing battle on the field reinforcing hegemonic discourses of what is to be a Pacific man.

### *Working with masculinities – cultural empowerment for men through sport*

> People know the reputation of Samoa and these kids eventually turn out to be great football players, good students and just. **Everyone wants [to be] one**.
>
> Rich Miano (emphasis added), University of Hawai'i Assistant Coach Football (Polynesian Power 2005)

Recent years have seen increased attention being given to 'the Pacific in global sport' (Uperesa and Mountjoy 2014, p. 263), with a growing number of Polynesian professional players joining the American National Football League (NFL) and Polynesian and Melanesian players joining the Australian National Rugby League (NRL).

The success of Pacific athletes in professional sports such as the NRL and NFL, and their contribution to pre-game war dances such as the haka, can inadvertently reinforce negative, or at least limiting, tropes of Pacific masculinity. Pacific sporting success is often accounted for in terms of Pacific men being natural athletes, fuelling the 'brawn' versus 'brain' discourse that portrays Pacific men as lacking foresight, having a poor work ethic, and not possessing the acumen for 'careful thinking' said to be required by more gentlemanly sports such as cricket (Coakley et al. 2011). The hypervisibility of Pacific men as 'big' and aggressive within Rugby League and National League Football renders their other attributes invisible.

Sport is seen by many as having an important role to play in addressing social issues and tackling inequalities, and Pacific communities' engagement in sport acts both as a social bridge for marginalised and disconnected Pacific communities, and as a tool for cultural diplomacy (Grainger 2006, 2009; Hokowhitu 2004). In Australia, the governing body of the National Rugby League endorses the potential of sport to effect social change and raise awareness of the broader cultural struggles affecting Pacific communities. But the National Rugby League also argues that to bring about change athletes themselves must first be willing and able to take on the role as leaders and cultural brokers for the Pacific communities they represent.

In an attempt to build players as 'people of character' and address the often-damaging masculinities present in and off the field, National Rugby League in Australia developed the Wellbeing and Education Programme (NRL n.d.). The programme includes professional development training for staff and athletes to explore respectful relationships, issues of mental health, social responsibility, alcohol management and the use of illicit drugs by players. In line with this vision, National Rugby League has designed a specific programme to educate Pacific athletes and the industry on the importance of understanding, engaging and developing Pacific cultures within rugby league. One way in which this has been achieved is through Pacific Cultural Leadership camps where players deemed as emerging leaders come together to reconnect with heritage and history and develop their leadership as Pacific Islander athletes (see NRL n.d.). Providing a safe space in which Pacific athletes can *talanoa* (dialogue, story) and safely unpack their vā-connections, feelings and thoughts can meaningfully support their success and life journeys (Fa'avae et al. 2021; NRL 2022).

Most recently in 2022, the Australian National Rugby League announced the establishment of a Pasifika and Maori Players Advisory Group and a Pacific Wellbeing Advisory Group, to foster the use of Pacific knowledge frameworks and systems by players and managers (NRL 2022). The aim was to build cultural safety in the industry and support athletes to achieve their athletic and academic potential. Efforts are being made to help athletes gain the skills and qualifications needed to progress into leadership and administration roles after retirement. Former National Rugby League player, Joe Galuvao, who is of Samoan heritage, provides an example of an athlete who has come through this particular pathway. He attended the 2012 NRL Pacific Cultural Leadership Camp before he retired in 2013 but went on to work as the National Rugby League One Community Program Manager, disrupting the stereotypical view that Pacific Islanders are only good as players on the field. The activities within the National Rugby League Wellbeing and Education program provides an opportunity for former Pacific athletes like Galuvao to support the next generation of young athletes through culturally responsive strategies that focus on cultural and spiritual strengths linked to collective leadership and continuity. Similarly, the Australian NRL is working across the Pacific region to promote and affirm respect for gender, inclusion and sexuality diversity.

Through the work of the National Rugby League, a path has been made available for the geographic and socioeconomic mobility of Pacific people. Sports-related movement builds on the earlier migration trends of Pacific people in the diaspora, but is unique in some ways because it not only affords media visibility but also provides economic rewards that far exceed those associated with other forms of migration, including a direct link to upward mobility via college degree programmes (see Uperesa 2014).

National Rugby League provides a means by which Pacific men in the diaspora are able to navigate the socioeconomic deprivation and mental health concerns they face within their communities. Although NRL may also reinforce hegemonic masculinities stressing physical strength and bravado, perceived as desired qualities in Pacific men, current initiatives such as the Pacific Cultural Leadership camps attempt to counter and disrupt such stereotypes, drawing on expertise within through key role models such as Nigel Vagana and Joe Galuvao. National Rugby League provides a unique space to effect positive social change and provide meaningful education for Pacific male athletes and their communities in Australia (and elsewhere), by attempting to break down some of the stereotypical and societal barriers that undermine marginalised groups. Pacific male athletes have a responsibility to act as cultural brokers for their communities, being in a position of power and leadership both in sport and in their local communities. The importance of generous and understanding male role models who value vā and vahaloto relationships, particularly for first and second-generation Pacific communities, is central to cultural empowerment, the preservation of cultural continuity, and language change within the diaspora.

## Conclusion

Dance and sport provide important spaces in which Pacific men are countering hegemonic discourses and disrupting mainstream portrayals of Pacific men and moana masculinities. The spectacle of the dance stage and the sports field provides only one of many portrayals of Pacific masculinity. Efforts to disrupt mainstream and hegemonic theorisations of masculinities using vā and vahaloto place Pacific worldviews at the centre. They encourage Pacific men to show meaningful leadership in ways that heal, narrates and expresses a range of moana masculinities well fitted for the challenges that lie ahead.

## Notes

1 In this chapter, we use the term moana to encompass the Pacific Ocean or the Blue Continent as well as the continents of Australia and North America.
2 Polyfest is the largest Polynesian secondary school festival in the world. Since it started in 1976, Polyfest has grown and it is a space in which high school students are able to showcase their cultural identities and language through traditional dance, songs and chants.
3 A concept in the Gagana Samoa (Samoa) and Lea fakaTonga (Tonga) languages mainly.

## References

Aleke-Fa'avae, I., Bourke-Jackson, L., and Pilisi, A.S., 2021. Exploring savageness and Niue Takalo. [Webinar]. Tagata Pulotu Seminar Series – Tupumaiaga a Niue Trust and Unitec Pacific Centre. *Youtube.com*, Nov 23. Available from: https://youtu.be/uj_p3pJWAJQ [Accessed 9 August 2022].

All Blacks Experience, 2022. History of haka. *All Blacks Experience* [online]. Available from: https://www.experienceallblacks.com/insider-information/haka/history-of-haka/ [Accessed 21 July 2022].

Anae, M., 1997. Towards a NZ-born Samoan identity: Some reflections on "labels". *Pacific Health Dialog*, 4 (2), 128–137.

Anayo, J., 2017. *Transnational identities in a digital age: A case study of Niue*. PhD thesis, RMIT University.

Atutolu, S., 2020. Keke Boy [song]. In *That's Me, That's Team*. Independent.

Cadzow, J., 2013. The quiet one. *The Sydney Morning Herald*, April 30. Available from: http://www.smh.com.au/rugby-league/league-news/the-quiet-one-20130421-2i948.html [Accessed 21 July 2022].

Coakley, J., Hallinan, C.J., and McDonald, B., 2011. *Sports in society: Sociological issues and controversies*. 2nd ed. New York: McGraw Hill.

Fa'avae, D.T.M., Tecun, A., and Siu'ulua, S., 2021. Talanoa vā: Indigenous masculinities and the intersections of indigeneity, race, and gender within higher education. *Higher Education Research & Development*, 41 (4), 1075–1088. doi:10.1080/07294360.2021.1882402

Fehoko, E., 2016. Pukepuke Fonua: An exploratory study on the faikava as an identity marker for New Zealand-Born Tongan males in Auckland New Zealand. In: N. Hadjigeorgiou (ed), *Identity, belonging and human rights: A multi-disciplinary perspective*. Leiden: Brill, 113–124.

Gibbs, P., 2016. Men's matters: Changing masculine identities in Papua New Guinea. In: A. Biersack, M. Jolly, and M. Macintyre (eds), *Gender violence & human rights: Seeking justice in Fiji, Papua New Guinea and Vanuatu*. Acton: ANU Press, 127–158.

Grainger, A., 2006. From immigrant to overstayer: Samoan identity, rugby, and cultural politics of race and nation in Aotearoa/New Zealand. *Journal of Sport and Social Issues*, 30 (1), 45–61. doi:10.1177/0193723505284277

Grainger, A., 2009. Rugby Island style: Paradise, Pacific people, and the racialisation of athletic performance. *Junctures: The Journal for Thematic Dialogue*, 12, 45–63.

Halter, N., 2015. *'To see with their own eyes': Australian travel writing on the Pacific Islands c.1880–1941*. PhD thesis, The Australian National University. Available from: https://openresearch-repository.anu.edu.au/handle/1885/155964 [Accessed 26 July 2022].

Hamley, L. and Grice, J.L., 2021. He kākano ahau–identity, Indigeneity and wellbeing for young Māori (Indigenous) men in Aotearoa/New Zealand. *Feminism & Psychology*, 31 (1), 62–80. doi:10.1177/0959353520973568

Hokowhitu, B., 2004. Tackling Māori masculinity: Genealogy of savagery and sport. *The Contemporary Pacific*, 16 (2), 259–284.

Hokowhitu, B., 2014. Colonized physicality, body-logic, and embodied sovereignty. In: L.R. Graham and H.G. Penny (eds), *Performing indigeneity: Global histories and contemporary experiences*. Lincoln and London: University of Nebraska Press, 273–304.

Hokowhitu, B., 2016. Monster: Post–Indigenous studies. In: A. Moreton-Robinson (ed), *Critical indigenous studies: Engagements in first world locations*. Tucson: University of Arizona Press, 83–101.

Jolly, M., 2008. Moving masculinities: memories and bodies across Oceania. *The Contemporary Pacific*, 20 (1), 1–24. doi:10.1353/cp.2008.0010

Mackley-Crump, J., 2015. *The Pacific festivals of Aotearoa New Zealand: Negotiating place and identity in a new homeland*. Honolulu: University of Hawaii Press.

Macpherson, C., 2004. From Pacific Islanders to Pacific people and beyond. In: D. Pearson, P. Spoonley, and C. Macpherson (eds), *Tangata Tangata: The changing ethnic contours of New Zealand*. Auckland: Thomson Dunmore Press, 135–156.

Moreton-Robinson, A., 2016. Introduction: Locations of engagement in the first world. In: A. Moreton-Robinson (ed), *Critical Indigenous studies: Engagements in first world locations*. Tucson: University of Arizona Press, 3–16.

Moseley, C., 2010. *Atlas of the world's languages in danger*. Paris: UNESCO

Muliaumaseali'i, M., 2017. *The space in-between: an ethnographic study of mobile technology and social change in rural Samoa*. PhD thesis, RMIT University.

Ng Shiu, R., 2011. *It's like going to the moon: The experiences of Samoan tertiary health students at the University of Auckland*. PhD thesis, University of Auckland.

Nosa, V., Adams, P., and Hodges, I., 2011. Distinctive alcohol cultural practices amongst Niuean men living in Auckland, New Zealand. *Kotuitui: New Zealand Journal of Social Sciences Online*, 6 (1-2), 62–72. doi:10.1080/1177083X.2011.592198

NRL, n.d. Wellbeing and education. *NRL* [online]. Available from: https://www.nrl.com/wellbeing-and-education/characterwise/about/ [Accessed 20 July 2022].

NRL, 2022. NRL launch Pasifika and Maori advisory groups. *NRL* [online], March 30. Available from: https://www.nrl.com/news/2022/03/30/nrl-pasifika-programs-launch/ [Accessed 26 July 2022].

One Wellbeing, 2021. The rise of Pacific Islander and Maori athletes in sport. *One Wellbeing* [online], July 29. Available from: https://onewellbeing.com.au/the-rise-of-pacific-islander-maori-athletes-in-sport/ [Accessed 20 July 2022].

Panapa, L. and Phillips. M., 2014. Ethnic persistence: Towards understanding the lived experiences of Pacific Island athletes in the National Rugby League. *The International Journal of the History of Sport*, 31 (11), 1374–1388. doi:10.1080/09523367.2014.924105

Pilisi, A.S., 2020. Negotiating service within areas of responsibilities: Experiences of New Zealand born Pacific tertiary students. Masters dissertation, Auckland University of Technology.

Polynesian Power, 2005. Directed by R. Pennington and J. Spear. USA: ESPN.

Pryke, J., 2014. *On the rise: Pacific Islanders in Australia*. The Australian National University, Canberra. Available from: http://devpolicy.org/presentations/2014-Pacific-Update/Day-2/Jonathan-Pryke.pdf [Accessed 26 July 2022].

Sai, A., 2007. *Tamot: Masculinities in transition in Papua New Guinea*. PhD thesis, Victoria University, Australia.

Spoonley, P. and Bedford, R., 2012. *Welcome to our world? Immigration and the reshaping of New Zealand*. Auckland: Dunmore Publishing Press.

Tagata Pasifika, 2020. Niue men lay challenge to elevate language. *Tagata Pasifika* [online], 8 December. Available from: https://tpplus.co.nz/community/niue-born-men-lay-challenge-to-elevate-language/ [Accessed 26 July 2022].

Talagi, F., 1982. Early European contacts. In Government of Niue and University of South Pacific, *Niue: A history of the island*. Suva: Suva Printing & Publishing Co, 111–120.

Tengan, T.K., 2002. (En)gendering colonialism: Masculinities in Hawai'i and Aotearoa. *Cultural Values*, 6 (3), 239–256.

Tengan, T.P.K., 2008. Re-membering Panalā'au: Masculinities, nation, and empire in Hawai'i and the Pacific. *The Contemporary Pacific*, 20 (1), 27–53.

Tengan, T.P.K., 2016. The mana of Kū: Indigenous nationhood, masculinity and authority in Hawai 'i. *New Mana*, 55.

Togiatama-Otto, P., 2019. Through my brown eyes: Niuean school boys' experiences in two New Zealand secondary schools. *SET: Research Information for Teachers*, 3, 12–18. doi:10.18296/set.0147

Uperesa, F.L., 2014. Fabled futures: Migration and mobility for Samoans in American football. *The Contemporary Pacific*, 26 (2), 281–301.

Uperesa, F.L. and Mountjoy, T., 2014. Global sport in the Pacific: A brief overview. *The Contemporary Pacific*, 26 (2), 263–279.

Vilitama, M., 2015. *On becoming a liquid church: Singing the Niuean 'Fetuiaga Kerisiano' on a distant shore*. PhD thesis, Charles Sturt University.

Wendt, A., 1996. Tatauing the post-colonial body [online]. *Span*, 42–43, 15–29. Available from: www.nzepc.auckland.ac.nz/authors/wendt/tatauing.asp [Accessed 26 May 2022].

Williams, M., 2018. *The ASB Polyfest: Constructing transnational Pacific communities of practice in Auckland, New Zealand*. PhD thesis, University of Auckland.

Young, K.M., 2017. Masculine compensation and masculine balance: Notes on the Hawaiian cockfight. *Social Forces*, 95 (4), 1341–1370. doi:10.1093/sf/sox022

# 12 Making meaning out of objects: Self, connectedness and belonging among sexuality diverse men and transgender women in Papua New Guinea

*Ruthy Boli-Neo, Jamee Newland, Angela Kelly-Hanku, Herick Aeno, Peter Aggleton and Kerry H. Robinson*

## Introduction

Historical, anthropological and other ethnographically-informed research has long documented the role that material culture plays in shaping human life in past and past and present societies, including gendered and sexual lives. Coming to value the role that matter and materiality play in 'meaning-making,' and in recognition of the fact that non-human objects have not been given due prominence in studies of this process, a 'new materalism' has developed in sociology and cultural studies. This has triggered new efforts to make sense of the way in which material objects, in the form of the mundane objects that people, families and societies interact with, experience and use in everyday life, mediate human culture and relationships (O'Toole and Were 2008). Such objects include clothing, body ornaments, cooking utensils, agricultural tools, books and other written documents, ceremonial objects and more. They may also include children's toys, mobile phones and computers, medical equipment and musical instruments. The meanings attached to these and other objects varies across people and communities, as well as over time, as does the way in which their use moderates and gives rise to our social world.

Objects as possessions are symbolic of a person's identity and as such can be used to signal who people want to be, how they want others to view them, and group belonging. They may also speak to broader issues of religion, class, gender, sexuality, citizenship and consumption. Examining and making sense of these objects within a specific cultural framework provides important insights into understanding the social lives of the people and communities to which these objects belong (O'Toole and Were 2008). Gaining access to and understanding of the cultural meanings and the value of material objects within social contexts involves both listening to narratives and considering how objects are used performatively. Here, the word 'narrative' refers to the stories people tell about these objects, both at individual and societal levels, as a way of talking (and thinking)

DOI: 10.4324/9781003142072-15

about their lives, experiences, values and cultures (Woodward 2007). But objects are also performative in that people engage and interact with them, actively influencing how an object is constructed and the meaning/s it communicates (Woodward 2007). Understanding the narrative character and performativity of objects in the contemporary Pacific requires us to look closely at the relationships between people, places, and things — a process which enables deeper understanding of the cultural, social, economic and political relations present within specific places and the differences between them.

Anthropologists and archaeologists, as well as traders, missionaries and colonisers, have long been engaged in the acquisition (through exchange, appropriation, theft or otherwise) of material culture across the globe, but particularly in socities deemed 'primitive' or Other. Papua New Guinea has long been such a site. Much of the attention given to material culture in Papua New Guinea has focused on historical and cultural items from the past (Craig 2005), such as sculptures and masks (Eves 2009), rock art (Lamothe 2008; Byrne 2013; Llamazares 2013), and stone carving tools (Hardy and Sillitoe 2003; Torrence 2011) as well as *tapa* cloth. Tapa in particular has also ignited interest through its contemporary use in moderating personhood, and Christian practice (Adams and Thomas 2013; Hermkens 2015; Barker and Hermkens 2016). To date this attention to material culture has been almost entirely directed towards the analysis of cis-gender men's artefacts, with far less attention given to women's creations and creativity, with the exception of the recent documentation of pandanus textiles, such as mats, and *bilums*, handwoven string bags made and used by women as well as tapa inspired clothing and shoes (Bonshek 2010; Andersen 2015; Gnecchi-Ruscone 2017, 2019).

## *Gender, sexuality and material culture*

Human expressions and experiences of gender and sexuality are intimately connected to material objects and vice versa. For example, unlike in other contexts where museums, galleries and historical research are beginning to showcase the experience of being transgender, non-binary and sexuality diverse (Adair and Levin 2020), little to no attention has been given to the material culture(s) of gender, sex and/or sexuality diverse individuals and communities in Papua New Guinea. Informed by anthropological research as well as by renewed interest in the material turn in the social sciences and humanities, in this chapter we reflect on the narrative and performance associated with four everyday objects to reflect on what these tell about kinship, gender, sexuality and belonging for sexuality diverse men and transgender women in Papua New Guinea today.

As part of a larger project to expand our understanding of sexuality diverse men and transgender women in Papua New Guinea beyond a focus on the limited confines of illness and disease, we undertook a life history project. By the term 'life history' (Dhunpath and Samuel 2009) we mean a qualitative study of experiences over the life course through interviews (Kelly-Hanku et al. 2021;

Aeno et al. under review) using a visual object biographic approach. This work required participants to share stories about an object or artefact of personal value and significance. Our focus on objects which carried strong personal and social meanings stemmed from the desire to understand the lived experience of sexuality diverse men and transgender women, whose stories are generally rendered invisible or dismissed. In this sense our work is political. The aim of the project was, through storytelling, to challenge some of the stereotypes that prevail concerning gender and sexuality diversity, by providing alternative narratives of lives rooted in individuals' own experiences and perspectives.

The project was conducted in the nation's capital – Port Moresby – and six other provinces (Central, Morobe, Milne Bay, Western Highlands, Simbu and Eastern Highlands). Participants came from 14 different provinces, reflecting the four geographically and culturally diverse regions of the country. Despite this diversity, these regions are similar in that they are predominately socio-culturally patriarchal and heteronormative. Understandings of being male or female are framed within binary perspectives of gender perceived to be determined by biology. Heteronormative practices, such as marriage, are expected if not socially compulsory. Participants in the study self-identified as transgender women, gay men, men who have sex with men, heterosexual and bisexual. One participant did not identify with any particular gender or sexuality category.

Participants brought a variety of artefacts to include as part of their stories. They included photographs of important people in their lives; medicinal and decorative plants; condoms; bottles of HIV antiretroviral therapy; clothing; modern and traditional bodily ornaments, such as ear and hand rings, leg and arm bracelets and necklaces; mobile phones; music players; and the Bible and other books (see Figure 12.1 for a collage of objects). Each of the objects held a

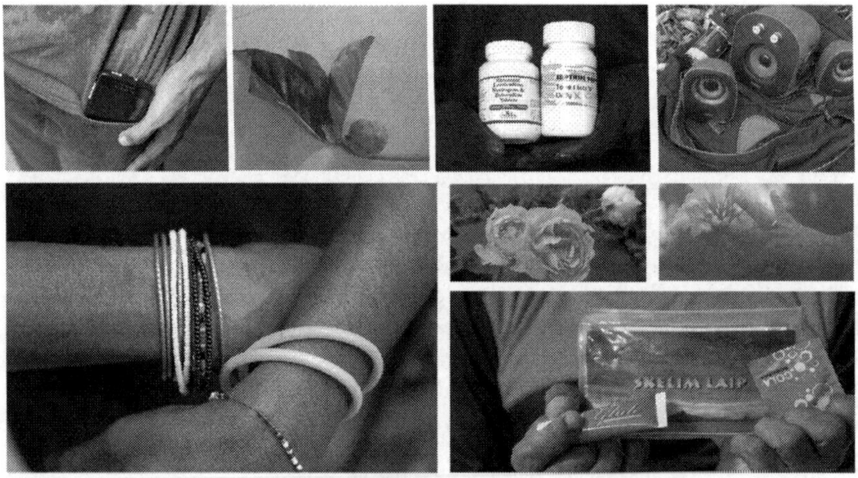

*Figure 12.1* Collage of objects.

special meaning for the person concerned, speaking in a sensual, tactile, material and embodied way to the social life of the owner. We use four examples of the objects shared by participants (identified by a pseudonym) that speak to the importance of relationships, kinship and family relatedness, and self-identity and rights that were described as culturally significant for those individuals concerned.

## Object biographies

### *Booklet: 'I always put my faith in this book. It looks at our rights'*

Describing himself as a 'normal boy' who socialises with 'real' boys, at the time we met him Luwis was was a 28-year-old man from a mountainous region in the central highlands of Papua New Guinea, Simbu Province. Although he had sex with both men and women, he identified as 'straight.' He first had sex with women in his early twenties and, following a short prison sentence of 18 months for a crime he did not reveal, he came to know first-hand about sex between men. Luwis recalled prison as a place in which sex between men was an everyday occurrence, motivated by violence, group membership, revenge and the need for protection. Within the prison walls, he recalled there being little room for pleasure, desire or sexual attraction, a story not uncommon in closed settings (Kelly-Hanku et al. 2015). Having served his sentence, Luwis moved to the coast and made his home in an urban settlement in Lae. Although sex in prison was remembered as anything but pleasurable, after being released he sought the freedom to have sex with anyone he wanted, including, but not exclusively with men, secretly. Had he stayed in his home province Simbu, he feared shame and violence brought about by transgressing cultural norms of heteronormativity and not fulfilling the cultural expectations of marriage and starting a family.

When we met and asked Luwis about his object of importance, he presented us with a copy of the booklet (see Figure 12.2) that he received when, after leaving prison, he joined Kapul Champions, a Papua New Guinean non-government organisation which promotes the rights of sexuality diverse men and transgender people. The booklet is entitled *Are you a man who desires other men? Are you a transgender person? Do you know your rights?* and has a cover image depicting someone dressed in the traditional attire of the Gahuku people of Goroka, Eastern Highlands Province. The booklet provides information about sexuality and gender diversity and HIV in the country. It also gives the contact details of organisations available to address the legal needs of sexuality diverse men and transgender people.

Having broken the law and served time in prison, the law (and Papua New Guinean constitution) took on an important and new role in Luwis' life. It was perhaps no surprise that we first came to meet him at a legal literacy training meeting organised for members of Kapul Champions[1]. Hearing about our interest in the life histories of people like himself, Luwis approached us to be interviewed. The booklet, distributed throughout the country, was important to

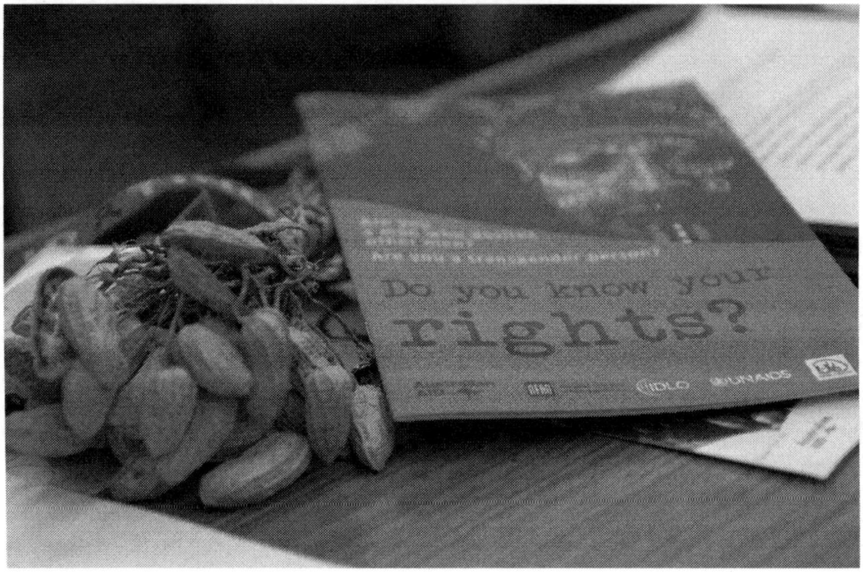


*Figure 12.2* Booklet.

Luwis because, as he said, 'It includes people like me.' Inclusion and representation thus speak to the exclusion and absence of representation Luwis, and no doubt many others, feel from mainstream Papua New Guinean society.

'I always put my faith in this book,' said Luwis. Carrying the booklet in his bilum, he took it with him wherever he went: 'It looks at our rights, those people like us. I don't just carry it around, whenever I'm around, I sit down and read it.' Reading the booklet provided the information Luwis lacked in understanding his sexuality, including the Western sexuality terms and labels used by Kapul Champions and others. It also helped Luwis to further understand his rights, such as fair and equal treatment by community, family and service providers. The book was also symbolic, communicating to Luwis that he was not alone in his efforts to explore sexuality and rights, a journey he was entitled to make in a patriarchal and masculinist society. Despite the book providing Luwis with the knowledge of rights and sense of belonging, he believed he could not express his sexuality openly and freely for fear of violence and discrimination.

### *Conch shell necklace: 'It's a sign of strength and courage'*

Remembering her childhood with fondness, Apsi, a 33-year-old transgender woman from the Central Province, recounted growing up behaving like a girl and playing and spending time with girls (Kelly-Hanku et al. 2021). Apsi described being called *tolevavine* at this time, which is a local name in her mother's vernacular given to men trapped in a woman's body. Apsi spoke of growing up in her mother's village surrounded by other tolevavine, many with whom she had familial ties. Recalling the stigma and discrimination she had experienced at school (Aeno et al. under review) and in public places, made Apsi reluctant to express who she was to others in public places. This changed when she went to university where she felt proud to freely express herself. Later in life, Apsi describes living with HIV as a double stigma, but a stigma that she has tried to overcome.

Relatedness and family kinship are important parts of social life in Papua New Guinea. For Apsi, they were characterised by strong bonds and positive relationships with family, and she described them as critical in her ability to overcome life challenges. Kin relationships provided Apsi with the support to be courageous and to have the strength to be who she was. She explained her courage as coming from her mother, elder sister and elder brother – family who were described as her 'backbone because they've always told me, live the life as who you want, who you choose to be.'

Apsi's object of value was a shell necklace (see Figure 12.3) that was a gift received from her mother in 2011 before her mother passed. Apsi held up the necklace so that we could see its detail; it was made from small conch shells that were threaded together using nylon cord. Slowly moving between each shell, Aspi described how the necklace was a symbol of strength, explaining that she not only wore the necklace to remind her of her mother, but also like a 'Catholic rosary.' Apsi explained that each shell in the necklace had a special message and meaning, signifying each challenge she had conquered or overcome over her life as a

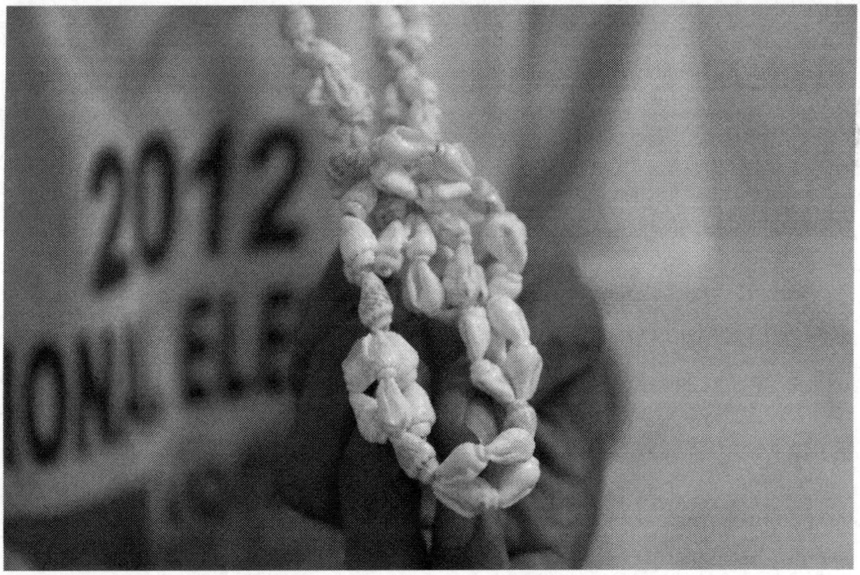


*Figure 12.3* Conch shell necklace.

transgender woman and also as a person living with HIV. For Apsi, the necklace communicated its prestige and status, reminding her of her strength.

The value of the necklace was also from the act of giving – a present from her mother. This gift was a loving memory of how caring and loving her mother had been and was able to fulfil a cultural practice of respecting the dead by keeping the object for years. Apsi also explained how the spirit of her dead mother still strengthened her and she therefore treasures and keeps the necklace in remembrance of her mother to motivate her to be strong and be who she chooses to be. For Apsi, the necklace embodied kinship support for gender diversity and represented support and strength – giving hope of fair treatment irrespective of gender identity, sexual orientation or ethnicity.

### *Photograph of friend: 'I have nothing that is important, apart from my living objects that are my friends'*

Born in Milne Bay Province, a largely matrilineal society on the south-eastern coast of Papua New Guinea, Wilfred was a 31-year-old man who identifies as gay. Early in his life Wilfred moved from the coast to Goroka, the capital of the Eastern Highlands Province, where he lived with his mother and sister and had little contact with his biological father – a time he described as 'fun' since he felt free to explore feminine dress and behaviour. When Wilfred was 13 years old his mother remarried, but his new stepfather could not accept Wilfred being transgender as a child, or his interest in other men as he grew up. Wilfred's 'transgressions' were met with violence. Having cared for his mother until her death from cancer, Wilfred took her demise as the opportunity to leave a home filled with violence.

Trying to settle in other cities, Wilfred finally set up home in Goroka. Throughout much of this time there, Wilfred was subjected to significant community-based violence including hate speech, physical violence such as being stabbed, and tragically on his 21st birthday, violently raped by a group of men. Searching for a safe place to live, Wilfred was finally taken in and adopted by a family from Simbu Province living on the outskirts of Goroka town. The mother in this family was younger than her husband, was open to Wilfred's difference and others like him and persuaded her husband to accept him into their home. At 25, Wilfred therefore found himself in a new and much more loving family. In recognition of his belonging, and because terms such as 'gay' were at that time still not widely used in Papua New Guinea, he was given the *tok ples* name from the province (Simbu) his adopted family came from — *Amaku,* or light skinned woman. As a coastal person, he was fairer than most highlanders and he described his gendered habitus and performance as feminine; this name only being used within the family setting was thus fitting. And although Wilfred's dress was feminine and 'girly,' he identifies as gay, not transgender. While accepted, Wilfred was still expected to conform to custom and traditional values regarding sex and marriage, albeit with a twist. As he was not yet married or committed to another man, he was forbidden to bring men home.

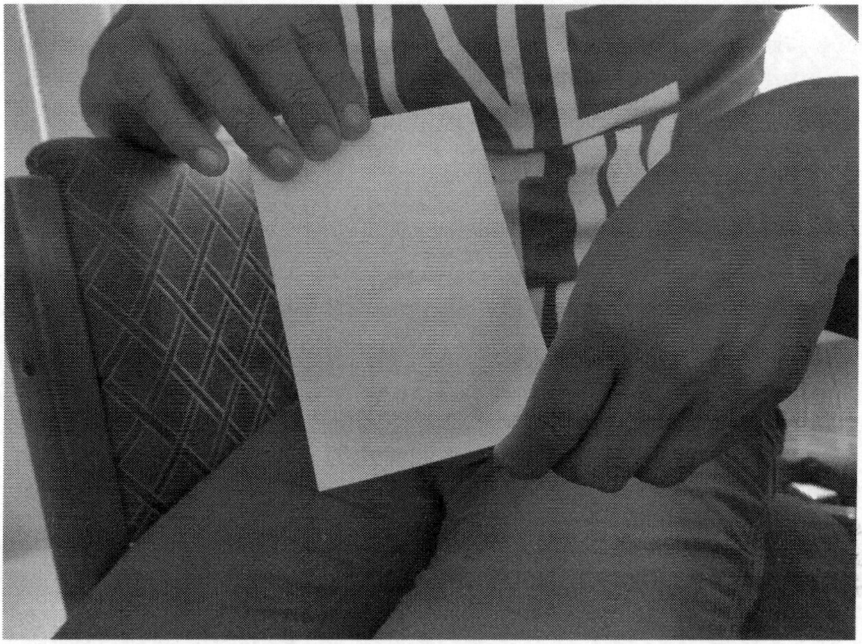

*Figure 12.4* Photograph of friend.

Wilfred spoke of a life of dislocation and disconnection from important social relationships as result of his mother's death and ongoing violence. In turn, this experience made him value the social relationships he has with his friends, as illustrated in the material object he shared: a photograph of a gay friend (see Figure 12.4). Never a sexual partner, this friend has been a significant mentor and role model to him. While the photograph is a material object, his friend — his real object — is a human one. When speaking about this friend, and the photograph of him, Wilfred said, 'I don't value anything that I have in my house like a TV.' Indeed, he said he has 'nothing that is important, apart from my living objects: that is, my friends.' Describing these friendships as living objects and recalling his friendship with the man in the photograph, Wilfred spoke of the enduring and tolerant nature of his friend's support: 'He was always there. I've put him through shit to get over what I had to get through.' This photo, and the friend within it, reminded Wilfred of the potential others could see in him, even when he himself could not. Speaking of the importance of friendship in his life, he shared how friends would comfort, support and stand up for him – literarily and figurately wiping his tears away. In doing so, these friends 'could put stones for you to step on and put bridges for you to go over. Even if you cut the bridge and fall, they will not let you fall; they will pick you up and tell you to go on. The road is there, they showed me and said it's mine to claim.'

Human objects depicted through photographs communicated the importance of social relationships and belonging for Wilfred, but it was Wilfred's life history and his description of the photograph that transformed it from the blank image shown to the reader, to a shared story (Hoskins 1998), revealing much about Wilfred's life of social disconnection and violence. Relationships, represented as 'bridges to walk on,' had provided him with a safety net and a sense of belonging. Wilfred's human objects, his friends, accepted him for who he was, and the photo served both as a visual representation of courage and hope and a reminder that as a gay man, he was deserving a fair treatment, acceptance and opportunity.

### *Bras: 'A bra is important to me because I don't have breasts'*

After leaving her birth family and village in Morobe, Alberta moved to the nation's capital. At the age of 26 when we first met her, she was living above the bar she worked in, hosting nights where members of her community and their supporters could come and enjoy drag show performances. Never dressing as a boy, Alberta was always happiest when dressing like other girls. Indeed, she was one of the few transgender women we met in the study who went by a woman's name and always presented herself in typically Western feminine dress. During her formative years her community of birth had accepted and supported her; indeed, it was her community that changed her male name and assigned her the female one she continued to use with some pride. Alberta sometimes identifies as a transgender woman, but not always; at other times she is simply a woman.

While in her childhood, Alberta had found acceptance of her gender identity (Kelly-Hanku et al. 2021), beyond her birth community and in later years, her being transgender, particularly with respect to her clothing and makeup, resulted in repeated stigma and discrimination. Alberta recounted experiences of discrimination at school including being forced into and locked in the boys' toilet at school (Aeno et al. under review). Not fitting in influenced Alberta to look for social relationships beyond the school environment. In Port Moresby, she made friends with sex workers in night clubs, people who would introduce her to the economic potential and promises of sex work. Her experiences of school-based stigma and these new social relationships and understanding of sex work, influenced Alberta to leave school by the time she was 14 years old. At 17, she moved to Port Moresby, the capital of Papua New Guinea, where she continued to live and advocate for respect and justice for transgender people until her untimely death with HIV in 2016.

Sitting in the room above the night club where she worked, rented for her by one of her expatriate boyfriends (a client), Alberta surrounded herself with material objects of femininity: decorative jewellery; women's clothing; shoes; wigs; lipstick; face powder; mascara and other items used to dress herself for work. But of all these objects, the ones that mattered most to her were her bras (see Figure 12.5). Noticeably wearing a black bra, Alberta described how she filled her push up bras using 'a little bit of tissue.' Since she did not have her own breasts, by birth or through feminising hormones, finding ways to feminise her

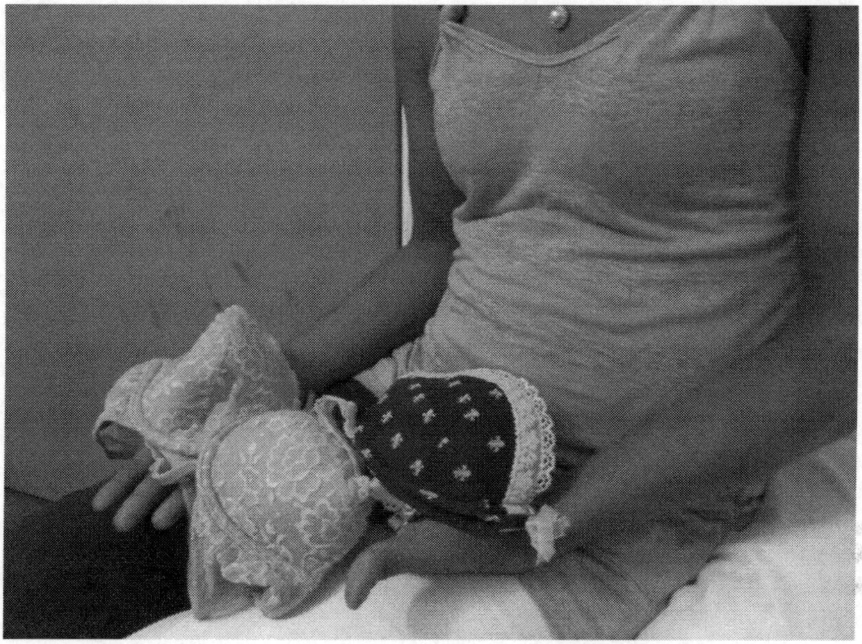

*Figure 12.5* Bras.

body mattered to her. Her bra was symbolic and transformative because it made it visibly possible to express a type of femininity she desired.

Alberta deeply desired to have her own breasts. Several years prior to our meeting, Alberta had travelled overseas to Thailand to participate in a regional meeting of transgender women. In the hope that she might develop more permanent breasts while in Thailand, she accessed hormone therapy. However, upon her return, in the absence of ongoing hormone treatment and the professional care needed to oversee her use of hormones in Papua New Guinea, or the money to continue to access it from overseas, Alberta had no other option but to discontinue therapy. But as we spoke, her dreams of both having breasts and undergoing sex reassignment surgery remained strong. Alberta's happiest moments in life were bound within family and kinship, a place where she was supported to express her true gender identity and 'happy to stand up and tell the whole world that my parents love me, and I am happy to be a woman. I wear my breast[s] in front of my mum and dad and that is the happiest thing in my life. I've got my family support.'

Clothing may be viewed as an object of everyday life, but for Alberta, clothing was transformative (Lyttleton-Smith and Robinson 2019). Her bra was a performance negotiated through feminine clothing practices (Hourigan 2015) that was more than modesty or functioning – it was the relationship between Alberta and her bra that embodied, defined and communicated relevant gendered performance (Entwistle 2000). For Alberta, a bra both functionally and symbolically communicated a complex array of information about who she was as a woman – both to herself and to others. Her bras were also bound up with acceptance of gender embodiment, facilitating connectedness and belonging to her gendered self (Young 2005) among family and kin, and in wider social life. This acceptance was particularly important for Alberta who lives in a country where those who transgress the culturally inscribed forms of gender performance expected of them, face social and legal discrimination (Herdt and Poole 1982; Kelly-Hanku et al. 2020; Kelly-Hanku et al. 2021).

## Concluding remarks

As in other parts of the world, the material culture of Pasifika people tells important stories about lives and culture. While documentation of material culture in Papua New Guinea has typically focused on valuable and traditional non-human objects, such as stone tools (Hardy and Sillitoe 2003) and tapa cloth (Hermkens 2015), this chapter has begun the documentation of the material culture, of other less visible Papua New Guineans. Across the diverse objects shared by participants in this study, various themes emerged, including the importance of relationships, kinship and family relatedness; love, self-identity and courage; and human rights, justice and health. Within each of these themes, issues of visibility and belonging were prominent.

These material non-human objects, some of which represented significant people, provide new insights into the lives of these Papua New Guineans who are frequently framed in public discourse as being at risk of sexually transmitted infections such as HIV and a risk to the morality of heteronormativity. At face value, these shared objects may be seen as mundane – dull, unexciting and lacking in perceived value – they are not the objects usually found in ethnographic exhibitions of Pasifika cultures. But in participants' discussion these objects took on a social life above and beyond their functionality; communicating self-acceptance and care, and representing future aspiration and potential. They also spoke to the importance of family, kin and community, embodied inclusion, connection and belonging. The objects and the stories they convey stand in stark contrast to those typically talked about in relation to sexuality diverse men and transgender women in Papua New Guinea. Making meaning out of objects, they speak of self, connections and belonging – universal themes that connect these people and their communities to their land and to others.

## Note

1 The Papua New Guinean peer-led civil society organisation representing men of diverse sexualities, originally referred to as MSM (men who have sex with men) and transgender people.

## References


Adair, J.G. and Levin, A.K., 2020. *Museums, sexuality, and gender activism*. Abingdon: Routledge.

Adams, J. and Thomas, N., 2013. *Tapa: Barkcloth paintings from the Pacific*. Birmingham: Ikon Gallery.

Aeno, H., et al., Under Review. Memories of school among sexuality diverse men and transgender women in Papua New Guinea. *Gender and Education*.

Andersen, B., 2015. Style and self-making: String bag production in the Papua New Guinea Highlands. *Anthropology Today*, 31 (5), 16–20. doi:10.1111/1467-8322.12200

Barker, J. and Hermkens, A.K., 2016. The Mothers' Union goes on strike: Women, tapa cloth and Christianity in a Papua New Guinea society. *The Australian Journal of Anthropology*, 27 (2), 185–205. doi:10.1111/taja.12193

Bonshek, E., 2010. Collecting relations in Melanesia: making a contemporary collection in the Western Highlands of Papua New Guinea. *Journal of Museum Ethnography*, 23, 7–20.

Byrne, S., 2013. Rock art as material culture: a case study on Uneapa Island, West New Britain, Papua New Guinea. *Archaeology and Physical Anthropology in Oceania*, 48 (2), 63–77. doi:10.1002/arco.5004

Craig, B., 2005. What can material culture studies tell us about the past in New Guinea? In: A. Pawley et al. (eds), *Papuan pasts: cultural, linguistic and biological histories of Papuan-speaking peoples*. Canberra: Australian National University, 493–513.

Dhunpath, R. and Samuel, M., 2009. *Life history research: Epistemology, methodology and representation*. Rotterdam: Sense Publishers.

Entwistle, J., 2000. Fashion and the fleshy body: Dress as embodied practice. *Fashion Theory*, 4 (3), 323–347.

Eves, R., 2009. Material culture and the magical power of dance objects. *Oceania*, 79 (3), 250–262. doi:10.1002/j.1834-4461.2009.tb00063.x

Gnecchi-Ruscone, E., 2017. The extraordinary values of ordinary objects: String bags and pandanus mats as Korafe women's wealth? In: A.-K. Hermkens and K. Lepani (eds), *Sinuous objects: Revaluing women's wealth in the contemporary Pacific*. Canberra: ANU Press, 151–179.

Gnecchi-Ruscone, E., 2019. Bilum, bilas, bilumwear: PNG women loop stylish dresses to create new identities. *ZoneModa Journal*, 92 (2), 47–69. doi:10.6092/issn.2611-0563/9961

Hardy, K. and Sillitoe, P., 2003. Material perspectives: Stone tool use and material culture in Papua New Guinea. *Internet Achaeology*, 14. doi:10.11141/ia.14.3

Herdt, G.H. and Poole, F.J.P., 1982. 'Sexual antagonism': The intellectual history of a concept in New Guinea anthropology. *Social Analysis: The International Journal of Social and Cultural Practice*, 12, 3–28.

Hermkens, A.K., 2015. Mediations of cloth: Tapa and personhood among the Maisin in PNG. *Oceania*, 85 (1), 10–23. doi:10.1002/ocea.5070

Hoskins, J., 1998. *Biographical objects: How things tell the stories of people's lives*. London: Routledge.

Hourigan, S., 2015. *Expressive materialities: Clothing, reciprocal appearance management and the mother-daughter relationship*. PhD thesis, Griffith University.

Kelly-Hanku, A., Aggleton, P., and Boli-Neo, R., 2020. Practical justice as an innovative approach to addressing inequalities facing gender and sexually diverse people: A case example from Papua New Guinea. *Culture, Health & Sexuality*, 22 (7) 822–837, doi:10.1080/13691058.2020.1736633.

Kelly-Hanku, A., et al., 2015. Sex, violence and HIV on the inside: Cultures of violence, denial, gender inequality and homophobia negatively influence the health outcomes of women and men in closed settings. *Culture, Health & Sexuality*, 17 (8), 990–1103. doi:10.1080/13691058.2015.1020877

Kelly-Hanku, A., et al., 2021. Gender diversity among 'boys' in Papua New Guinea: Memories of sameness and difference in early childhood. *Children & Society*, 35 (1), 144–158. doi:10.1111/chso.12408

Lamothe, D., 2008. Striking out into the interior: Travel, imperialism, and ethnographic perspectives in The Autobiography of an Ex-Colored Man. In: *Inventing the New Negro: Narrative, Culture, and Ethnography*. Philadelphia: University of Pennsylvania Press, 69–90.

Llamazares, A.M., 2013. A semiotic approach in rock-art analysis. In: I. Hodder (ed), *The meanings of things: Material culture and symbolic expression*. London: Taylor and Francis, 271–277.

Lyttleton-Smith, J. and Robinson, K.H., 2019. 'I like your costume': Dress-up play and feminist trans-theoretical shifts. In: J. Osgood and K.H. Robinson (eds), *Feminists researching gendered childhoods: Generative entanglements*. London: Bloomsbury, 61–84.

O'Toole, P. and Were, P., 2008. Observing places: Using space and material culture in qualitative research. *Qualitative Research*, 8 (5), 616–634. doi:10.1177/1468794108093899

Torrence, R., 2011. Finding the right question: Learning from stone tools on the Willaumez Peninsula, Papua New Guinea. *Archaeology in Oceania*, 46 (2), 29–41. doi:10.1002/j.1834-4453.2011.tb00097.x

Woodward, I., 2007. *Material culture, narratives and social performance. Objects in contexts*. London: SAGE.

Young, M., 2005. *On the female body experience: Throwing like a girl and other essays*. North Carolina: Oxford University Press.

# 13 Localising human rights for men of diverse sexuality, transgender women and people living with HIV in Papua New Guinea

*Emmanuel Peni and Tim Leach*

Emmanuel Peni (Manu) is a Papua New Guinean activist from Wewak in the East Sepik and is prominent in several of the country's social and environmental justice movements. He works regionally and globally, but it is his expertise in Papua New Guinean social justice movements that brings him to this conversation in this chapter, particularly his presidency of *Kapul Champions*, Papua New Guinea's national community organisation for men with diverse sexualities (MDS) and transgender women. I (Tim Leach) am an old community-sector worker from Sydney, Australia who has worked in HIV and queer community movements in Australia and elsewhere, off and on, for more than 20 years. I have worked a lot with *Kapul Champions* and *Igat Hope*, Papua New Guinea's organisation for people living with HIV. Manu and I decided to write this chapter together as a conversation, a *talanoa* as many others in the Pacific would say, following many, many other conversations over decades of collaboration. Most of our work has taken place within that highly dynamic space in which sex, sexuality, gender, HIV and human rights intersect. Like so many of our conversations, this one meandered back and forth, sometimes to unanticipated destinations.

We talk about human rights and how we see – Manu from within, myself from outside – Papua New Guineans making sense of these rights, interpreting and shaping them for local use. Both *Kapul Champions* and *Igat Hope* promote human rights for particular communities, whose members identify – at least at some times or to some degree – in respect of HIV status, sexuality or being transgender, so our discussion of rights necessarily involved issues of identity. Indeed, any analysis of human rights in Papua New Guinea requires a focus on identity. It is precisely because of the way Papua New Guineans conceptualise and prioritise their identities, that human rights are being localised, or indigenised, in the country.

Our chapter explores the appropriateness, or otherwise, of dominant framings of human rights, particularly with respect to sexual diversity and transgender women, but also as applied to people living with HIV in Papua New Guinea: the country provides an interesting case study for the examination of these issues as they are experienced across the Pacific because Papua New Guinea has the Pacific's largest

DOI: 10.4324/9781003142072-16

population of people living with HIV and has no tradition of a third gender, unlike several neighbour states such as the Samoa, Tonga and the Cook Islands (see, e.g., Veukiso-Ulugia et al. Chapter 3; Futter-Puati Chapter 4.).

We draw upon two primary sources of evidence. First, there is Manu's lived experience, from his insights grounded in a lifetime at the heart of human rights struggles in his country of birth, and as a non-heterosexual man heading up a movement of men with diverse sexualities. Second, we draw from Tim's doctoral research on human rights movements in Papua New Guinea. Our chapter starts with issues of identity and moves on to perspectives on human rights, although we both agree that the one cannot be separated from the other in Papua New Guinea.

## Notions of sexuality and gender are shaped by time and space

Some truly excellent research has been conducted on Papua New Guinean male sexuality, sexual behaviour and gender non-conformity.[1,2] Many of these researchers and writers have explored the challenges of trying to understand Papua New Guinean gender and sexuality by reference to external, often Western, frameworks. I asked Manu how these phenomena in Papua New Guinea might be understood if temporarily freed of such frameworks. He began by saying:

> There are research reports by social scientists about sex, sexuality and gender in Melanesia. These reports are too few and not adequate to give a proper understanding. And again, often these reports were written by outsiders who may never fully understand the nuances of the cultural dynamics. In Papua New Guinea, there are some aspects of culture which have no definition. Additionally, these may not have words attributed to them, may never be mentioned, but are still acknowledged and considered an integral part of life of Melanesia.

Immediately, I wondered how outsiders like myself could ever write about non-heteronormativity if it involves phenomena that have no definition, to which no words can be ascribed, and which are never actually discussed. But Manu thinks we should not be put off by this and calls for more research to be done. And while he definitely thinks more of it needs to be done by Papua New Guineans, the perspectives of non-Papua New Guineans are also valuable: 'Outsiders' observations are crucial in being able to see and document what we, as Papua New Guineans, cannot see because of our blind spots,' says Manu. But he emphasises the critical importance of outsiders energetically interrogating their insider/outsider status when doing this work, as countless academics themselves have also advocated. Manu and I both see the value in insiders and outsiders working together on these issues – we like to think this chapter is an example of such collaboration, and as seen in other chapters in this book.

Manu explains that when men with diverse sexualities and transgender women from Papua New Guinean travel abroad and experience sex, sexuality and gender outside of their homes, they see something very different to their own experience at home. Even if what they see has appeal in this external domain, they do not necessarily try to import it, says Manu, or try to explore how these experiences can be defined, appreciated or expressed in Papua New Guinea. Manu calls them 'outsiders' understandings,' and while there may be some limited expression of these in Papua New Guinea, they are mostly concentrated only in what Manu calls 'safer spaces.'

This notion of space comes up repeatedly in our conversation. Manu talks about the spaces (or contexts) that exist in Papua New Guinean life and which contextualise and thereby give meaning to everything, including sexuality and gender, but he also talks about spaces that are created in *response* to sexuality and gender identity. When he talks of these safer spaces, he means larger population centres such as the national capital of Papua New Guinea, Port Moresby, or Lae, the provincial capital of Morobe, a large shipping port and the country's second-largest city. But he also uses safe spaces to refer to safe mediums such as text messages between individuals, reports with limited readerships or conversations with restricted audiences. Manu continued

> I see so much male sexuality in Papua New Guinea that is fluid. I also see that gender can also be fluid in Melanesia. And so, identity and expression are subjected to space and time. They occur on a continuum and can't be allotted into compartments, do not occur in neat little boxes such as LGBTIQ+[3]. These tags are misleading and continue to label individuals. By doing so, these compartments cause individuals to stick out like a sore thumb. Two diverging experiences are lived by individuals labelled (either by others or by themselves). Some articulate these clearer definitions and labels by being confident about themselves, protect themselves better, understand themselves better and are of happier disposition. This is the good thing about how outsiders and their labels shape the understanding and lives of Melanesians in Papua New Guinea. The negative consequences of taking up these labels are that they can bring a false sense of security, unwarranted and unrestrained pride, disrespectful flamboyance and a demand for human rights without any form of responsibilities.

There is quite a lot in this observation. Manu makes important points about the fluidity and essential contextualisation of Melanesian sexuality, at least in so far as the constituents of *Kapul Champions* are concerned. I heard these same points in the research interviews I conducted between 2015 to 2017, and the theme has been explored by many others. In their introduction to a collection of reflections on non-heteronormative people in the Pacific, Besnier and Alexeyeff (2014) write about the fluid, contextual nature of Pacific sexuality and gender identity, noting there are different stories to be told about the same non-heteronormative person depending on where they are at the relevant time.

Manu makes the same point: the identity a non-heterosexual man or transgender woman from Papua New Guinea might assume in Sydney or London is different to the one they live in Port Moresby or their village. He says,

> We are submerged into the gay culture there. We begin to acquire some habits and exhibit stereotypical behaviours. For us in these countries, being gay becomes central. There is the security, sex, comraderies, friendship and more – a community, communal feeling within the LGBTIQ+ community. When we are in Papua New Guinea: Family, Community, Tribe and Clans become our Centrality. We have sex, for sure, but do not experience the community and organise around that community.

People who have worked in HIV will be very familiar with the almost unavoidable pressure exerted by the global response to compartmentalise communities with reference to risk. We have been encouraged to put both others and ourselves in boxes – as people living with HIV, gay, men who have sex with men (MSM), sex workers, and so on – so that we can work out how to keep us/them safe by delivering the tailored programmes we/they apparently require. And yet a person living one identity in one place and a second (or third) elsewhere frustrates efforts to compartmentalise. This is the reality for many of the people with whom Manu and I have worked. I found this same resistance to compartmentalism in my research, and at multiple levels. For example, *Kapul Champions* constituents frequently identify as a man with diverse sexualities in one setting and a transgender woman elsewhere. I asked Manu about this, and he reiterated that, for many of the organisation's members, gender is fluid, defies description and is contextual: 'The expression of this gender is limited to a time and a space,' says Manu. And yet, despite the difficulty in ascribing words to these states and expressions, '… these are elaboratively displayed in artefacts, paintings, cultural marks and totems and dutifully expressed in poetry, singing and dancing, music, jokes and satire.'

Manu wants us to understand how gender and sexuality might be described and expressed in ways other than through words, and how these other forms of expression may serve as ongoing records of the ways in which communities have accommodated, absorbed or even celebrated non-heteronormative states of being. But at some point, I think, attention has to turn back to the words and expressions that *are* used. All the people I interviewed in my research, who were largely living in Port Moresby and connected to the movements I studied, had been regularly compartmentalised through the use of Western terms, and most had been on the receiving end of harshly verbalised descriptions of their sexuality or gender identity, with vilification, discrimination and violence being very common experiences. Transgender women, in particular, had been subjected to very harsh treatment.

Manu had more to say about compartmentalisation:

> The issue is when a word is attributed to the behaviour or the state. When a researcher says it's 'gay' or 'bisexual,' then the interpretation by different people will differ. Perhaps, ten years from now, even Papua New Guineans who are not in tune with their culture will see it from an outsider's point of view and say, *it's gay*, when the sexual activity was perhaps really an

> expression of a phase, of love, of fulfilling a sexual need, of establishing power or of kindness from one to another. It is probably the interpretation of the act and the word used to describe it that could mislead.

Manu is wary of labels generally, and of the tendency to interpret behaviour as identity in particular. The risks of applying Western categories to non-Western sexualities and genders have been noted by many others (e.g., Boellstorff 2011). Manu sees multiple risks here: first, behaviours get explained as identities, and second, Papua New Guineans who are assigned (or self-assign) these labels are encouraged to behave in ways that offend. Manu explained his observation: 'trans women or trans men are part of the population but are never labelled or differentiated or singled out,' but many transgender people interviewed through my doctoral research told a very different story, saying that they were indeed singled out and mistreated for their expression of transgender identity. Manu replied,

> In many villages outside of Port Moresby, there are transgender men and transgender women. They are not defined by their behaviour or gender expressions. They are defined by how they relate to their families, communities and clans and the greater environment – Melanesian Spiritualism. They are treated just like everyone else. They are called by their names and understood by reference to how they are related to a family clan, never by their expressed gender or sexuality. Transgender people in cities like Port Moresby and Lae are experiencing the clashes in cultures – identities as driven by outsiders, development narratives and aid programs. By these identities, they become isolated, disconnected and therefore are not connected to the Melanesian Spiritualism. Therefore, they may experience harassment.[4]

Manu asks us to think about how global notions and movements are understood within Papua New Guinea, and to then move from this big picture to consider the smallest of spaces (again, this notion of space) – conversations in small groups, text messages and the like, where a person can be one identity while living a different one elsewhere. I wondered how much choice people really had over the choices they made about identity and expression, and the degree to which this choice is constrained by the need for safety. This notion of a safe space was a common theme in my earlier research, which documented high levels of discrimination and violence, including sexual violence, perpetrated against men with diverse sexualities, transgender women and people living with HIV. The people I interviewed often considered their experiences to have been impacted by location: 'cities are safer but there is no acceptance in the villages' (the exact opposite of Manu's view); 'the coast is much safer than the Highlands'; and 'I am safe in my village but as soon as I step outside of it, I am at risk.' They also talked about safe places in the sense of social groups: 'I am safe in my community but not when outside'; and 'I am safe with my other MDS and transgender friends.'

Hanuabada, a traditional Motuan village within Port Moresby, is often referenced as a kind of combination of these two safeties – renowned as being a place where queer families have been constructed in an accepting community (see the short 2018 film *Guavas and Bananas: Living Gay in Papua New Guinea*). Interviewees who were people living with HIV commonly talked of the safety to be found by being with other people living with HIV, the value they placed on their community of HIV-positive *friends* (a term used between people living with HIV, and which can be used as a kind of code to protect the confidentiality of HIV status), and the critical importance of drop-in centres and other places where people with HIV can gather in safety. However, these safe spaces were being conceptualised by interviewees for my research, they felt they could behave as they wished within them, even live a different identity if they chose. Some, mostly people living with HIV and men with diverse sexualities, could live a different identity outside of these spaces because their HIV status or sexuality need not be disclosed. By contrast, many transgender women did not feel they had this option and, where forced from these safe spaces, most just felt unsafe (and indeed *were* unsafe, given the high levels of violence to which they were subjected).

I remind Manu that people can get very agitated by discussions of identity. We talk about how it has meaning for sexuality and gender expression in many Western cultures, where people may actively assert an identity and take steps, sometimes quite dramatic steps, to have it recognised and acknowledged by others. Manu tells a story about a villager he knows who was born anatomically male but who lives as a woman. The villager is just being himself (Manu continues to use male pronouns for the villager), expressing his gender in the way that feels right for him. He isn't using his gender expression as an 'identity,' he just lives as he feels, says Manu. The villager does all the same kind of work in the community that is associated with men but otherwise lives and presents as a woman. From an outsider's point of view, it might be concluded that the community completely accepts him. He gives respect, he gets respect. It's how it has always been in Melanesian culture, thinks Manu.

I ask Manu how he sees himself and how that shapes his identity. He tells me:

> When I think of the word 'identity,' I begin with my name, and then I think of existing within a community, relating to other people. I see myself within the context of that community and my identity is shaped by what is around me. And then there is the physical expression of that identity. The Manu in Port Moresby is different to the Manu in Wewak, who is different to the Manu in the village – my lifestyle choices will be different depending on where I am, my sexuality will be managed differently, to the point that it's not a clear or forceful or irresponsible outward expression. I do not have to force myself to make these changes, I just do, and the transition is easy and seamless. When I am in the village, I am a villager, doing all the stuff that men in the village do. I am never making these changes because I am scared but because it is just the right thing to do, the respectful thing to do, and the right way to embrace the leadership role I am expected to take on. You give respect, you get respect.

I put to Manu that I have heard many, many stories of men with diverse sexualities and transgender women experiencing hurtful, horrible discrimination in many areas of public life, and that many have been vilified, excluded, persecuted and subjected to violence. Their lived experience has not been characterised by the respect to which Manu so commonly refers. Manu wonders about the role those individual men with diverse sexualities and transgender women may have played in those situations and whether assertive claims of identity may have contributed to negative responses. In asserting identity, did they give respect to their communities, he asks. I have heard this argument before, that the person experiencing discrimination bears some responsibility for it in that they have not shown respect or not met their own responsibilities. Yet the interviewees in my doctoral research demonstrated a deep understanding of the links between rights and responsibilities, and clearly articulated their responsibility to express their sexuality and transgender identity in respectful ways, and to manage HIV status responsibly. Many interviewees told stories of the efforts they went to show respect to their communities, and yet they were still subjected to stigma and discrimination in multiple forms.

There are multiple aspects to this story, of course. In asserting identity in ways that are out of keeping with the Melanesian community – such as adopting strategies commonly used in Western countries, using human rights arguments to assert individual entitlements and organising, in a political sense, around sexuality, gender and HIV status – the constituents of *Igat Hope* and *Kapul Champions* are doing something new, something which might be considered disrespectful to community, at least by some. But it might also be said that, in vilifying and discriminating against members of their own community, for matters as unimportant as HIV status, sexuality and gender expression, those who do the discriminating are also acting out of Melanesian character. I challenged Manu's suggestion that the people I interviewed might in some way have contributed to their predicaments or to the treatment to which they were subjected. Manu replied

> It is like me going to Australia and not trying to fit in. I must try to fit in because of the culture there. I must have a sense of myself and assimilate into the Australian culture. It's the same for me assimilating and living here as a Melanesian gay man, within a respected organised way. If a straight man has two wives and drinks and is promiscuous, then he is frowned upon. If a gay man becomes promiscuous and is loud and disrespecting an organised way of life, he or she must also be frowned upon. We must identify as a member of a community, family and the land – first and foremost. We have identified ourselves within this cosmology. I am we; I am a Papua New Guinean and I live as Manu in ways I honour my land and its life. I operate within this belief and organised system.

## Human rights frameworks that make sense in Papua New Guinea

Manu really challenges the external, outsiders' compartmentalising of sexuality based on risk. It fails to recognise the reality of Papua New Guinean life, he says.

But it also complicates the way in which human rights are understood and experienced in Papua New Guinea . When we're talking about human rights, we mean the freedoms and protections guaranteed to all human beings by virtue of the Universal Declaration of Human Rights and various international covenants. Many of these rights are also guaranteed by the Papua New Guinea constitution. Manu points to the discourse on sexuality and risk and how this same discourse invokes human rights frameworks as a means to protect the rights and interests of those communities deemed to be 'high risk.' Manu argues that this ends up linking, in the community's mind, human rights with culturally inappropriate categorisations of sexuality and gender, and then with disease and risk of death. Clearly, this is unhelpful, he says, and I agree. He sees HIV programme specialists as among the worst users of this flawed approach.

How depressing it is that the human rights of people living with HIV, men with diverse sexualities and transgender women have been associated with risk, disease and death. The idea of 'human rights' should be uplifting, and a reading of the Universal Declaration of Human Rights or the Papua New Guinea Constitution, with all its beautiful guarantees of human rights, should lift and inspire. But the way we so often approach the promotion of human rights in Papua New Guinea has the potential to unintentionally taint them. To begin with, there is an emphasis on negative rights (Parker 2010), which sees human rights advocacy focused on redressing rights violations rather than positive social reform. In consequence, the conversation around rights becomes a conversation around protecting those who are 'different' from the dominant culture and, inevitably, the conversation takes on an 'us versus them' tone.

In my research, I encountered strong resistance to this conceptualisation amongst interviewees, finding amongst them a far more nuanced understanding of their human rights. As many have observed, human rights in Papua New Guinea cannot be separated from sociality and community (see Lepani 2015), and work in Papua New Guinea has shown that human rights advocacy only really makes sense to people living with HIV, men with diverse sexualities and transgender women to the degree that it acknowledges the priority that people place on community connection. Constituents of *Kapul Champions* and *Igat Hope* reject human rights advocacy strategies that 'protect' them from the community by emphasising their otherness. But in rejecting these common articulations of human rights, the individuals concerned offer an alternative construction of their rights, one that celebrates community connection and that acknowledges the interrelationship of rights and responsibilities in Papua New Guinean community life. In this way, human rights are localised (Merry 2006a, 2006b, 2011), indigenised by people living with HIV, men with diverse sexualities and transgender Papua New Guineans[5] who craft human rights frameworks that emphasise the critical importance of Melanesian sociality and the interconnectedness of all things. Manu describes this interconnectedness as follows:

> Papua New Guinea, and the greater Melanesian society, sits on a complex web of relationships. Everything and everyone is connected to one and other. No one is excluded. Irrespective of sex, sexuality and gender. Everyone is connected to a family, clan, tribe, village, communities of all sorts, the plants and animals, other man-made items like canoe, axe or lifeless objects such as stone, wind and the sun. Everyone is connected to spirits of the land, oceans, rivers and the universe. The Melanesian names given to a child also connect Papua New Guineans to those who have departed, their ancestors and those who are yet to arrive to this world and those who are present today. All these relationships with varying degrees of connectedness mean no one is excluded. This is Melanesian Spiritualism.

Just as a Papua New Guinean's sexuality and gender can be understood only in context, it is the same for a person's human rights. These rights make sense only in so far as they are considered with reference to family and community. This is why the interviewees who shared their stories with me in my earlier work resisted some elements of the human rights framework they felt was being promoted in PNG. They did not like those elements that pitched one group against another. They did not like conceptualisations of human rights that failed to recognise the responsibilities Papua New Guineans have towards their families and communities. They did not like the approaches that demanded accommodation of their otherness, preferring conceptualisations that promoted inclusion and community. But a critical point here is that, while they may not have liked these common articulations of human rights, they placed great value on their human rights per se. They could critique these common framings of human rights while seeing that *better* human rights arguments, more appropriately framed, could lead to a better world for people living with HIV, men with diverse sexualities and transgender Papua New Guineans.

Manu sees the roots of contemporary dilemmas, such as the homophobia and transphobia to which *Kapul Champions*' constituents are subjected, to lie in Papua New Guinea's colonial past, with colonialists having brought two negative forces to Papua New Guinean life. First, they brought a new rigidity to compartmentalising and labelling of sexuality and gender, reinforced with religious instruction, that designated some categories as good and others as evil, generated divisions where they had not previously existed. This, says Manu, ran counter to the Melanesian way: 'Melanesians weaved life into a complete real time living experience where everything flowed and had an explanation of being. Nothing was bad or nuisance but all had a purpose in life.' And second, they imported laws that penalised those who fell into the wrong compartment. These twin impacts continue to shape the thinking of Papua New Guineans and Melanesians: '… the articulation of what outsiders brought and continue to bring today continues to be the key points of argument used by colonised Papua New Guineans to defend their prejudice, their stigma, discrimination and hate.'

Manu points to a recent controversy in Papua New Guinea arising from the promotion of LGBTIQ+ causes by diplomatic missions. At the time we talked, the Australian High Commission and US Embassy had both (and separately) promoted queer equality on social media, specifically by posting on social media images of diplomatic staff posing with rainbow flags. These acts subsequently prompted some highly vitriolic abuse towards non-heteronormative Papua New Guineans and their supporters, particularly women (Fennell 2020). And so we see the hand of the colonialists in every aspect of this sorry story. The colonialists – working through both Church and State – introduced marginalisation and criminalisation of behaviours where this marginalisation and criminalisation did not previously exist. By doing so, they then provided the hate language to be used against those subsequently marginalised and criminalised. And in conducting the triggering event, outsiders precipitated the latest round of hatemongering, largely through the technology of social media.

If outsiders have caused the problem, it is best we do not exacerbate the situation by pushing for a human rights framework that is not fit for purpose. Manu returns to his earlier points:

> The other wave of outside influence is from those who promote Human Rights and related services for the LGBTIQ+ community in Papua New Guinea. While these people have the best of intentions, the act of defining, labelling with tag, attributing human rights to the members of this community and providing tailor-made services for them is already a setback. The act, the conversation, the discussions and service provision identifies, isolates and puts a red flag on an individual. This individual is marked right at the outset of this development intervention. Once this person is defined and tagged, this individual is now further removed from the connections to the family, the clan, the tribe and the communities. This person is now looked at from the perspective of this label, this reference point. This shines a light on the individual and thus the family, and so the families become more conscious, more aware of their relative's differences. Before this label and the service targeted for this individual, this person was an ordinary member of the family. Before this label by the outsiders, the family would not have treated the person with dismay, disdain, dislike, disrespect and with disapproval. The label causes the feelings and the subsequent negative reactions and treatment from the family. When the immediate family begins to disconnect with the labelled individual, then a rippling effect occurs whereby the neighbours, the communities and, eventually, members of the greater society do the same. This is what members of the LGBTIQ+ community are experiencing here today.

This is a very grim take, but it neatly signals the problems involved in common articulations of human rights: the ones that emphasise labelling of individuals as marginalised, that emphasise the otherness of those labelled and cause further disconnection between the person being labelled and that person's family and community. Manu summarises: 'Why all this labelling and naming and compartmentalising in order to give rights to people who already have them in communities?' This is why it is so important that human rights work is done differently, following the lead of those who have a much more positive view of human rights frameworks: men with diverse sexualities and transgender women embrace human rights frameworks that position them with reference to their families and communities, that promote inclusion, that acknowledge the interconnection between rights and responsibilities, that emphasise the importance of articulating their rights, not as special, but as the same as the rights enjoyed by other Papua New Guineans.

It is a problem that many development agencies continue to promote human rights frameworks that are not fit for purpose. We need trusted community organisations that understand what frameworks are most appropriate: organisations like *Kapul Champions* and *Igat Hope*.

## People living with HIV have their own stories

*Igat Hope* has a proud record of achievement over more than 20 years, in often extremely challenging circumstances, and no story of the epidemic in Papua New Guinea is complete without proper reference to this history. One of *Igat Hope's* contributions has been to document, and be a vehicle for the recounting of, experiences of stigma and discrimination of people living with HIV. These are, of course, different to the other experiences of men with diverse sexualities and transgender women in Papua New Guinea, but there are undoubtedly commonalities. An HIV-positive identity was voiced by many of those interviewed for my earlier research, and most interviewees reported experiences of discrimination linked to their HIV status. This discrimination was manifested in rejection by family, friends and communities; in unfair treatment across multiple domains of life including healthcare, employment and education; in vilification and violence.

Many interviewees agreed that life is better for people living with HIV than it used to be, explaining how successful treatment had been in reducing community fear of HIV and enabling the compassionate and caring nature of Papua New Guineans to flourish. And yet, interviewees perceived these gains as fragile in nature and observed that HIV-related discrimination continues. People living with HIV recognised that the treatment they received from others disrespected their human rights. They demonstrated a solid understanding of their human rights. When asked what they understood their rights to be they were generally very able to rattle off a list of their most important rights. Most commonly, interviewees cited the right to employment/livelihood/engage in marketing or business; the right to movement (which was often described as the right to freedom from violence, as people living with HIV felt safe in some spaces but feared moving beyond those spaces would bring the risk of violence); the right to freedom of speech or expression; the right to health care, particularly non-discriminatory health care; the right to live free from stigma and discrimination; and the right to HIV treatment.

Here, people living with HIV conceptualise their rights as inseparable from their responsibilities. Many interviewees reflected on the additional responsibilities they bore as a consequence of their status, including to prevent transmission and to take treatments faithfully so as to ensure – and maintain public confidence in – their effectiveness. Interviewees talked about how easy it is for stories to be spread about their failure to meet these responsibilities and the fact that there were many more stories of these failings than actual cases thereof. But the frequency of these stories' telling is consistent with a keen understanding that rights and responsibilities are connected. Just as is the case for men with diverse sexualities and transgender women in Papua New Guinea, it is not uncommon for people to suggest the experiences of discrimination of people living with HIV are, in some way and to some degree, attributable to their own behaviour. And yet, through my research, and in the decades of work with *Igat Hope* that preceded it, I encountered countless examples of people living with HIV being subjected to discriminatory treatment where they were acutely aware of their responsibilities and seeking to meet them, had no desire to challenge cultural norms, and were not disrespecting community.

Manu has also done a lot of HIV work, and one of *Kapul Champions'* key goals is to prevent HIV transmission among its community and to provide care to those with HIV. But he prefers to leave it to *Igat Hope* to comment on HIV issues. Manu does note, however, the critical value to HIV prevention of understanding how Papua New Guineans see themselves in relation to their families and communities. He talks about how he does prevention work (for both HIV and COVID-19) by asking people to think about protecting their family and their obligations to their community. He laments some of the HIV prevention work that has been done by foreign aid agencies, often with vast sums, work that caused more fear, more uncertainty, more anger and more division: 'The family or relations – relating and connecting is very powerful, no amount of colonial law or western money can break the bond. In Melanesia, the currency is kinship, relationship and connections.'

The human rights terrain can sometimes be hard to navigate. On the one hand, communities are asked to grapple with things that may be perceived (rightly or wrongly) as new to culture; efforts are made to promote and protect people's entitlements to express identities or choose behaviours that might be considered new or external. At the same time, this needs to be done in ways that do not offend, that are experienced as respectful of culture rather than anti-culture, that draw on cultural elements to enhance messaging and shape behaviours. Outsiders might well wonder how on earth these tensions can be balanced. But one thing research has revealed is that the members of *Igat Hope* and *Kapul Champions* are less flummoxed by this tension than might be imagined. Individuals, families and communities have already worked out how to navigate these challenges, and how to work within culture to help it evolve in ways that will benefit their communities. Through their work, *Igat Hope* and *Kapul Champions* give voice to this knowledge. It is an example worth following, and the organisations should be properly resourced to support and lead.

The constituencies of *Igat Hope* and *Kapul Champions* have coalesced around notions of identity, encouraged by an international HIV response that tends towards categorisation based on risk, and to the ascribing of identities based on epidemiological categorisations. Perhaps it is not surprising then that Manu is so keen to explore and explain how he sees identity playing out in Papua New Guinea, particularly for these constituencies. Indeed, it is the way these constituencies are identifying with their larger families and communities that contributes so much to the localisation and indigenisation of human rights in Papua New Guinea.

## Notes

1 This chapter does not dwell on definitions of sex, sexuality and gender as they relate to men with diverse sexualities and transgender people in Papua New Guinea. 'Non-heteronormative' is a good catch-all descriptor although, in our experience, other terms are more commonly used in PNG. We use 'men with diverse sexualities' (or 'MDS') to include men who at least occasionally engage sexually with other men, including people the global HIV industry might be keen to describe as gay, bisexual or 'men who have sex with men' (MSM). Transgender members of *Kapul Champions* often use the term 'TG,' but we are using 'transgender' or 'trans men' and 'trans women' to describe people who may have been considered at birth to be of one biological sex but who, at least some of the time, live, identify or present with an alternative gender. Although, as we discuss in this chapter, the very act of naming and categorising brings problems.

2 Examples include the works of Herdt (2011), Knauft (2003), Stewart (2014) and Kelly-Hanku et al. (2021).

3 LGBTIQ+ is a shorthand descriptor for Lesbian, Gay, Bisexual, Transgender, Intersex and Queer. The descriptor is intended to encompass the diversity of non-binary, non-heteronormative identities and experiences. While Manu uses it, as this chapter will indicate, he is not necessarily a fan: a collection of labels is still a label.

4 Transgender women interviewed for my research were all living in Port Moresby, so Manu would say they all have experience of the clashes in culture that characterise life in urban settings.

5 See also work by Gibbs (2016) who described a layering of rights and culture in Papua New Guinea. And see Kelly-Hanku et al. (2020) who address issues of practical justice as another way to think about human rights and sexuality diverse men and transgender women.

## References

Boellstorff, T., 2011. But do not identify as gay: A proleptic genealogy of the MSM category. *Cultural Anthropology*, 26, (2), 287–312. doi:10.1111/j.1548-1360.2011.01100.x

Besnier, N. and Alexeyeff, K., 2014. *Gender on the edge: Transgender, gay and other pacific encounters*. Honolulu: University of Hawaii Press.

Fennell, J., 2020. Australian government accused of 'meddling' in PNG affairs after pro-LGBTQI social media post. *Australian Broadcasting Commission Radio Australia*, 28 May. Available from: https://www.abc.net.au/radio-australia/programs/pacificbeat/lgbtqi-catholic-png/12294792 [Accessed 12 April 2022].

Gibbs, P., 2016. Men's matters: Changing masculine identities in Papua New Guinea. In: A. Biersack, M. Jolly, and M. Macintyre (eds), *Gender violence and human rights: Seeking justice in Fiji, Papua New Guinea and Vanuatu*. Canberra: ANU Press, 127–158.

Herdt, G., 2011. Talking about sex: On the relationship between discourse, secrecy and sexual subjectivity in Melanesia. In: D. Lipset and P. Roscoe (eds), *Echoes of the Tambaran: Masculinity, history and the subject in the work of Donald F. Tuzin*. Canberra: ANU Press, 259–273.

Kelly-Hanku, A., Aggleton, P., and Boli-Neo, R., 2020. Justice as lived: Addressing the inequalities facing gender and sexually diverse men in Papua New Guinea. *Culture, Health & Sexuality*, 22 (7), 822–837. 10.1080/13691058.2020.1736633

Kelly-Hanku, A., et al., 2021. Gender diversity among 'boys' in Papua New Guinea: Memories of sameness and difference in early childhood. *Children & Society*, 35 (1), 144–158. 10.1111/chso.12408

Knauft, B., 2003. Whatever happened to ritualized homosexuality? Modern sexual subjects in Melanesia and elsewhere. *Annual Review of Sex Research*, 14 (1), 137–159.

Lepani, K., 2015. 'I am still a young girl if I want': Relational personhood and individual autonomy in the Trobriand Islands. *Oceania*, 85 (1), 51–62. doi:10.1002/ocea.5073

Merry, S.E., 2006a. *Human rights and gender violence: Translating international law into local justice*. Chicago and London: University of Chicago Press.

Merry, S.E., 2006b. Transnational human rights and local activism: Mapping the middle. *American Anthropologist*, 108 (1), 38–51. doi:10.1525/aa.2006.108.1.38

Merry, S.E., 2011. Measuring the world: Indicators, human rights and global governance. *Current Anthropology*, 52 (S3), 83–95. doi:10.1086/657241

Parker, R., 2010. Reinventing sexual scripts: Sexuality and social change in the twenty first century. *Sexual Research and Social Policy*, 7, 58–66. doi:10.1007/s13178-010-0004-3

Stewart, C., 2014. *Name, shame and blame: Criminalising consensual sex in Papua New Guinea*. Canberra: Australian National University Press.

# 14 Family and gender violence in Chuuk, Micronesia

*Manuel Rauchholz*

## Introduction

Life in the islands of Chuuk State, Federated States of Micronesia is characterised by ongoing, and concerning, issues of gender inequality and violence, masculinity, femininity and sexual exploitation (Smith 2014, 2019; Rauchholz 2016). A 2014 Federated States of Micronesia study reported that, among women, 33% had a lifetime experience of sexual violence, with 24% experiencing this violence within the last year. The same study also found that 35% of women who had experienced abuse did not report the violence to anyone (FSM Department of Health and Social Affairs 2014). Earlier research, amongst female college students in the Federated States of Micronesia pointed to similar experiences of sexual violence, with between 69% and 90% among the respondents reporting such violence (Rauchholz 2016). Subsequent research with men and women in four atoll island communities reinforced these figures concerning sexual violence, particularly as they affected young adolescent girl children (Rauchholz 2016). In small island communities, it is often only a handful of men who target women and girls in this way, ruining the reputation of all men, the majority of whom may never be involved in such actions. Research on violence, sexual abuse and exploitation in Chuuk shows that on average around 90% of the violence experienced is inflicted by a person's own family members, spouse or intimate partner (FSM Department of Health and Social Affairs 2014; Rauchholz 2016).

This chapter explores how the family is thought of and conceptualised within the larger social structure of Chuukese society and how incidents of violence are framed by certain cultural ideals as they relate to the everyday lived experience of women, young women and girls. The chapter defines violence as behaviour involving physical and verbal force or intimidation including unwanted physical touch. While important to be critically examined, the experiences of adolescent men, and men as the perpetrators and recipients of violence, are not engaged with here due to the limitations of space.[1]

## Family, gender and society in Chuuk State

Chuuk State comprises five geopolitical regions with three linguistically distinguishable languages. The islands are united by a shared interrelated *eyinang*,

DOI: 10.4324/9781003142072-17

matrilineal clan system, complemented by a secondary *éffékúr*, patrilineal clan system. Together there are over 40 identifiable clans which can trace connections and origins as far as Palau to the west and the Marshall Islands to the east, as well as to Kiribati to the south-east and Samoa in the far south (Goodenough 2002; Rauchholz 2010).

Historically, matrilineal clans comprised mothers, daughters, granddaughters and their (female) siblings and children (*inepwiineewu*) on collective land holdings centred around a hearth (*falang*) and meeting house/canoe house (*wuut*). These places and people formed a central part of a person's identity and sense of belonging. Hierarchy and rank were determined by order of settlement. Marriage relations were forged with people from another clan (exogamy), and on smaller islands where land resources were scarce cross-cousin marriage between two clans across multiple generations was common.

Ideally, the eldest men of a matrilineage or clan were the public face of the group. They were the spokespersons, chiefs, religious, political and military leaders and decision-makers of a group and represented or defended the interests of their clan, foremost the honour of their elders, 'mothers' and 'sisters,' with their lives. Sibling sets within one generation were and still are considered the building blocks of Micronesian societies (Marshall 1977) and sibling relationships are considered to be more important than marriage ties. Hence, fathers have played a secondary role in the raising of children. In urbanised settings not dependent on agroforestry and fishing but on wage labour (at home and more so abroad), family structures have undergone rapid change since the 1960s, with a stronger focus on the nuclear family, and as such, the father as the provider.

A trademark of kin relations is the idea and practice that kin share everything together. In a general survey of college students conducted in 2003, participants were asked to identify and rank the most important values in their society. 'Sharing' and 'sharing among relatives' were ranked as the most important values (Rauchholz 2016). In Chuukese, sharing or *aa fengen* literally means 'using/having/owning together,' which implies owning the same land and trees, and being together to share the food of the same land and from the same hearth. Thus, aa fengen forms the basis for secondary ideals that come from being of one shared substance in the form of *tipeewu ffengen* (unity of mind), *tong ffengen* (unity in love/compassion) and *angaang ffengen* (working together). Coming together around the hearth where food is prepared, and bringing together resources (money), minds and labour in unity around the (imagined) hearth is what signifies the ideal family since it sums up the Chuukese idea of the family as *inepwiinéew* (mother and sisters being one). The family unit then further extends outward to include the ties to the *eterekes* (direct lineages) and finally into the *eyinang* (clan) which forms the largest encompassment of the imagined family (see e.g., Goodenough 1951; Petersen 2009; Hezel 2013).

Within these three-tiered extended family units, a taboo on incest exists for siblings of the opposite sex and members of the same clan regardless of how distant their biological kin relationship may be. It requires that men not allude to, and must avoid, anything sexual related to the women of their family and clan, including classificatory siblings ('promised' brothers and sisters).[2] Ultimately, men are viewed as the guardians of the sexuality and dignity of their sisters, mothers and daughters. While there are contradictions and dangers to be negotiated, central to masculinity and male–female relationships is the perceived sexual drive of men, which is viewed as an innate force they can hardly contain by themselves. This drive is imagined as an unstoppable engine that can only be contained and controlled by the modesty of women and girl children. Cultural taboos of avoidance between men and their female kin therefore exist to contain (and therefore restrain) the sexual drive of men and boys (Goodenough 1949, 1951; Marshall 1983 [1981]).

In a matrilineal society, a daughter does not belong to the family of the father. As the father shares the same household as his wife, the danger and risk of breaking the sexual taboo is first with his own daughters and second with the daughters of his wife's sisters who may also be present in the same household. As the guardian of his wife and her sexuality, the husband occupies a conflicting or ambiguous role in traditional Chuukese society. As domestic living arrangements shift in line with a capitalist market economy model, past living arrangements cannot be maintained, nor can social distancing between fathers and daughters, and the classificatory brothers of the father, be maintained as they once were. If a man were to engage in any form of sexual relations with the unmarried female relatives of his wife living in his household this may be accepted or frowned upon, but not strictly speaking viewed as incest. So long as the person viewed as having initiated sex with the sisters or even the children of his wife or non-matrilineal dependents is still respected by the people of his wife's family and his own matrilineage, then these sexual behaviours may therefore not be censored by people from outside the kin group. Ideally, the brothers of the wife should actively step in, to challenge or even prevent the sexual exploitation of their sisters or younger girl children, but this often does not happen due to unspoken acceptance between men from both sides of a clan and with the tolerance of the elder women. Too many men and women alike do not see using physical force in a sexual relationship (such as between a man and a child) as an emotionally or physically harmful activity. Women and girl children are expected to absorb these abuses, and for many this is the accepted way of life.

When a senior kin member of status utilises his or her position for personal gain or sexual exploitation or shows violent behaviour towards more junior kin members, the people of his kin group will most likely avoid confronting him; he is taboo to them in this regard and essentially untouchable (also in the physical sense). His body, person and feelings are also attributed a higher 'market' value than those of the exploited or harmed junior members of the group. Persons of status, rank and wealth are also the public face of a family, lineage, kin group, village or political entity. As representatives of a kin group, their success and prestige are also the pride of the kin group they represent; both bestow honour upon each other and attempt to ward off shame and dishonour. Avoiding conflict and direct confrontation with the leader is part of showing proper respect and evokes respect from the wider community. Therefore, no action is taken to alleviate the situation of abuse or exploitation if the leader himself is engaging in sexual or violent acts not endorsed by his community of kin. One will likely continue behaving with respect towards that person to maintain a public face of 'harmony,' but in the minds of community members and behind the person's back there will be much gossip and expression of disapproval.

To respect a leader with humble obedience and servitude and maintain his honour and dignity in the public sphere is an essential part of the reciprocal relationship complex between kin in Chuukese societies, especially if the leader can provide well for the needs of his kin. This attitude of respect for a leader may at times work against a person who has experienced violence, rape or sexual abuse at the hand of a relative or the senior kin themselves. The harmed person and those who know what happened may not report the incident to a senior leader in their kin group or community out of respect for that person (that is, their father, uncle, or grandfather). To speak out would cause him and the family, lineage, and clan more harm than to keep quiet, as the leader would be expected to take immediate action that could even lead to the killing of the perpetrator.

In addition, the display of violence against a child, spouse or same-sex kin communicates a public display of ownership and belonging and a sincere interest in the doings – both public and private – of a child, wife or younger sibling. Displaying violence against a spouse can be aimed at warding off potential rivals who intend to coerce a married woman into a sexual encounter or relationship during her visit to another village or island. The husband's beating of his wife is meant to send a message to any potential rivals, and above all to his wife, that he will not tolerate any attempt by another man to compete and intrude upon the affection and sexual intimacy he shares and enjoys with his wife. The act of violence against his wife also signals the husband's willingness to fight with the same ferocity against any possible intruder. The same principle governs acts of violence against children or same-sex siblings when they are in violation of cultural norms and have displayed inappropriate behaviour deemed punishable. Sometimes the violence may be to ward off attacks by external persons who were harmed or for internal disrespect and violation of expected behaviour within the immediate family unit.

Having detailed the role that violence takes from intimate family relations to relations between families and individuals of different families and clans, I now turn to focus on the drivers of young women and girls' experiences of physical and emotional, even spiritual, victimisation that are associated with gendered cultural norms.

The underlying principle of masculinity in Chuukese society is that men are always on the lookout for an opportunity to have sex with a woman.[3] In response, young women and girls, and their mothers and brothers, always need to be on their guardto prevent this from happening. Chuukese people believe that men's sexual drive is a strong, natural force, and a central part of what it means to be a man. Allied to this force is a man's ability to flirt with, court and coerce women and girls into wanting to have sex with him. Love magic helps coerce a reluctant girl or woman to engage in a sexual relationship: 'Love magic is especially feared by women because the boundaries transgressed are both mental and sexual' (Dernbach 2005, p. 268). The real fears of the expected transgression of their bodies under the spell of love magic, with all the associated risks of a pregnancy outside of wedlock that could strip them of their dignity as a modest woman woman, was part of the mental drama, distress and trauma I witnessed through the high school aged girl friends of my three older sisters. It is difficult to capture and convey these emotions in an academic text.

At an early age, girls are taught three key lessons on how to prevent themselves from becoming a victim of love magic (Smith 2014, pp. 342–343): avoid talking back and reprimanding a man's advance thereby shaming him; avoid open rejection and taunting of a man's pursuits; and, humbly acquiesce to the verbal advances and try to quietly find a way out of the situation. Love magic is often used as a means of retaliation or revenge against a woman who has spoken harshly to a man in response to his advances (Dernbach 2005, p. 263; Smith 2014, p. 343). The threat of retaliation for rejecting a man's advances places young women and girls in a difficult position. Women are repeatedly harassed by men as they walk to school, go shopping and so on; however, they are always expected to respond in a quiet and humble way. If they humiliate or reprimand the harassing man in public, they can expect retaliation through love magic and scolding by their own kin in response to their behaviour. Women are expected to reflect behaviour that is the opposite to that of men. It is considered a cultural virtue for women and girls to quietly cope with and absorb experiences of aggression, violence, sexual harassment and exploitation, and many women encourage girls to take pride in this virtue (Smith 2014, 2019). By enduring pain and suffering they are, in their view, demonstrating moral superiority and fundamental female virtues as the harbingers of peace and harmony within their community.

In addition, men compete to be the first man 'on a woman' and, if successful, strive to leave their mark on the body of the woman as proof of their supreme masculine skills and sexual desirability to the opposite sex.[4] Women may also use love magic, but modesty prevents them from approaching men in the public sphere. Finally, physical force may also be used by a man if he were to encounter a woman or girl child walking by herself down a path or in the jungle, or find her alone in a house. To not take advantage of this opportunity for sexual activity might be viewed as 'wasteful.' Females should therefore never walk alone in Chuuk or be left alone in a house. To do so may be read by men as an invitation to sexual access to the lone female. In a modern urban Chuukese society on the capital island of Wééné, these kinds of masculine values pose a problem to female security (even in the home), mobility, education and business activity.

In summary, even during perpetration, women and men are expected to be discreet in these matters, avoid public conflict and be mindful of maintaining social distancing between male and female sibling sets to avoid anything remotely sexual as best they can. This extends to the point that a woman or girl will not enter a bathroom to go to the toilet if a male member of the family can see her enter. Likewise, men who want to be respectable will feel uncomfortable if they are put in a domestic situation where they can see fellow kinswomen entering a bathroom. As discussed next, culturally expected spatial distancing is difficult to maintain under crowded urban living conditions.

## Mobility between urban and rural settings

While Chuuk constitutes a discrete geographical and political place and space, it is also home to a people who maintain a high rate of mobility and interaction between their relatives and family members, between the rural and urban centres of their home islands, and between friends and relatives in the United States of America (USA) and its territories.

Chuukese islanders living in their urban island centres, in the USA and its territories are not able to easily maintain the social distancing culturally required between women and men of the same family or clan. Living spaces in urban island centres and in the USA are generally crowded. The only way a family can survive is to figure out ways to share the high costs of renting a home. A standard three-bedroom house might on average see three nuclear families sharing one bedroom each. To create some social distance, as girls enter puberty they may be relocated to the basement while boys entering puberty are moved to the garage to sleep at night whilst continuing to share toilets and showers in the home. In more extreme circumstances Chuukese boys may be relocated to another place, often wandering from one household to another.

The financial pressures in Chuukese families can be so dire that some families are forced to double the occupancy of the three bedrooms with one couple working night shifts while the other works day shifts. Since most Chuukese work in minimum wage jobs, this is the only way they can survive in costly places like on Oahu, Hawai'i. This overcrowding of living spaces, the movement to and fro of adults coming and going to work, children going and coming from school, and pre-school children being reared by their mothers, grandmothers, siblings, aunts and uncles in limited space, gives rise to heightened stress, often culminating in violence. Overcrowding and increased access to children and young adults of the opposite sex is sadly conducive to sexual violence and exploitation.

While elder female and male family members are at work and unable to provide social protection for girls at home, young girls become prey, as did one of my informants who shared how when she was a young girl, she and four other girls aged between 8 and 14 were regularly raped over a four-year period by a male member of the household, himself a teenager. Her story, she said, was no exception (Rauchholz 2016). Girl children and adolescent girls are often victimised by men within the communities or because of their own dependency on male heads of household granting them housing when they move from a rural to an urban setting. As much has been written about this situation (see, e.g., Smith 2014, 2019; Rauchholz 2016), the focus here will be on reverse mobility, which occurs when girl children or adolescents move from the urban US setting back to Chuuk, often a rural Chuukese setting. The reflections that follow are based on the experiences I have collected in the past few years from a number of young women who have returned to Chuuk and with whom I have spoken at length.

Their stories serve to illustrate some of the complexities not only of male-to-female but also female-to-female facets of the harassment, of verbally and emotionally violative behaviour a 'returnee' or a 'newcomer' might experience when returning 'home' from the diaspora.

## Consequences of mobility: 'Inside' experiences of family and community in the homeland

The advantage of interviewing Chuukese women who had returned to Chuuk as adolescents lies in their ability to reflect and articulate their experiences with an inside-outside comparative perspective. Their upbringing in the USA allows them to reflect more freely and critically on their sexualising and abusive experiences 'at home' in Chuuk. In most cases, life in the diaspora will have provided alternative options for living and being a woman. What follows are a few such recollections by young women who returned 'home' and who shared their experiences with me, as recently as 2022.

Sarah,[5] in her early twenties, did so in a conversation with Judy (see below). Sarah had returned to Chuuk at about the age of 14 and was working as an elementary school teacher at the time of our conversation when she shared the following:

> The most difficult part of the life as a teenage girl in Chuuk was the highly sexualised perspective of relationships between the male and female gender including the large amount of jealousy leading to gossip and among other things untruthfulness between our female relatives and friends. I would learn the hard way that even the slightest interactions between men and women were considered a sign of sexual interest, something I was not used to coming from my US school setting. There, guys and girls could just hang together without worrying about every word or action carrying the message of sexual interest. Over time I have mastered how to culturally disengage with men and yet I am still at constant risk of being sexually harassed on my way to school and even in the classroom while teaching. I can never feel safe.

Judy was a returnee to Chuuk and a female relative of Sarah (above). Having spent her first four to five years in Chuuk and then 10 years in the USA, she returned to Chuuk as a teenager and shared with me the following experience:

> I remember counting which of the men in the village around my age group had *not* inappropriately touched me. It came down to less than a handful. Part of it I always felt was my fault for spending time and engaging with them, while at the same time the boys I would spend the most time with weren't the ones who harassed me. It was often the ones that were just always around or randomly joined us wherever we went. So, it kept happening and people, including girls that were jealous of me, would think or gossip saying that I wanted it.

In her twenties now, Eva had lived in the USA for seven years before returning to Chuuk as a 15-year-old. She recalled

> The most 'memorable' experience I had was after I complimented a Chuukese man in his twenties. He had just scored us an impressive point in a volleyball game. I said his spike was good. I smiled at him while I said it. After the game some older women came up to me and asked if I would like for them to arrange a meet up to sexually engage with the man I had complimented on his volleyball skills. This was a frightening thought to my 15-year-old self, since it had not been my intention to sexually engage with anyone and certainly not with a man, I assumed to be far older than me, simply because he scored us a good point in the game. I thought he must have known I was underage and had in no way intended to indicate such interest over a compliment related to a game of volleyball. This experience would be the first of many and *was the least difficult to process out of all of them*. The spectrum of boys who would inappropriately touch me varied from children of 8 to men over 60. It happened so many times that I have forgotten many of the details and occasions, just the feeling of confusion, disgust, embarrassment and sometimes fear. Fear especially because I recalled an incident involving an older cousin who had also come to Chuuk from the USA and after going out with her paternal cousins to party was gang raped by them on the way home. There was nothing she could do about it. She did not want to bring disgrace to her father who was a respectable person in the community, so she just kept quiet and confided in me because of our shared bi-cultural experience in Chuuk and in the USA.

One of the biggest challenges for Chuukese young women raised in the diaspora but returning home to Micronesia derives from a clash of expectations – if not cultures. Some may lack awareness of the degree to which their gendered selves (as women) are sexualised in their homeland. In the USA, they were likely taught about the autonomy of their body, of having rights, and of girls being equal to boys and women being equal to men. They likely learned too about equal opportunity and experienced interactions in school and the workplace that were not overtly sexualised and/or segregated by the taboos and risks present in greater Chuukese society. They were also likely taught to articulate and voice their feelings and their opinions, argue their case and call out wrongdoings in violation of individually held rights, including bodily rights. Finally, they most likely learned to move freely by themselves to school and work without feeling at risk of being sexually violated in the way they do in Chuuk.

In consequence, Chuukese girls who have grown up in the diaspora testify that coming back to Chuuk can be one of the most challenging, yet most enriching experiences – enriching because they can meet the family members they have heard so much about, or talked to via Messenger or on Instagram; enriching too because they can finally see the ocean, islands, villages and homes of their parents, grandparents and extended family. But challenging when they see the simple living conditions and lack of education of their fellow kin, and challenging too when they experience the limitations of movement and expression imposed on young women in Chuuk. Some may fear returning in the first place because they anticipate the restraints that will be imposed upon them and the rebukes from family members when they do not behave as a 'home-grown' Chuukese woman or girl should. While men and boys may seek to violate them sexually, kinswomen may do so through slurs and gossip or by criticising and deconstructing the outspokenness and standards associated with their 'perfect' lives in the USA.

## Conclusion

Family relations in traditional Chuukese culture are ordered along matrilineal lines with patterns of behaviour understood and managed to prevent and protect women from male violence. The role of men in these family situations is viewed as that of guardians with responsibility for ensuring the safety of women and girl children living in their household. With economic and social changes to living arrangements in Chuuk, and abroad in the diaspora, these traditional arrangements have changed and with this there have been important consequences in male behaviour, with less protection afforded to women and girls as there once was. Increased mobility, including Chuukese travelling and living overseas brings new expectations of how men and women should interact, posing new challenges for the safety of young women and girls returning home to rural Chuuk. Finding ways to understand and address these tensions need to be an ongoing priority to ensure the ongoing safety of Chuuk women and girls caught between two cultures.

## Notes

1 Major publications on men and masculinity in Chuuk, Micronesia date back to the 1950s and 1970s and focus primarily on: male traditional roles (Gladwin 1953; Gladwin and Sarason 1953); values (Caughey 1977); violence and substance abuse (Marshall 1979, 1983 [1981]); and suicide (Hezel 1984, 1989). Many of the social problems associated with men were seen to be symptomatic of challenged male identities and the growing pains accompanying the emergence of new identities, given the fast pace of change in Micronesian societies at the time (Larson 1989; Hezel 1999, 2001, 2013; Marshall 2004). Aspects of masculine sexuality were first described systematically by Goodenough (1949, 1951), Gladwin and Sarason (1953), Swartz (1958) and to some extent by Rauchholz (2008, 2010). Moral (1996, 1998), Moral Ledesma (2000) and Dernbach (2005), to a limited degree, focus on the polar opposite of women's sexuality. Earliest reports though on male exploitations of female sexuality have been documented by Hambruch and Eilers (1936), Hanlon (1988) and Schlesier (1953).

2 Classificatory siblings are not siblings by blood or flesh but by social arrangement. A man and a woman may declare themselves a 'brother' and 'sister' thereby de-sexualising the relationship and allowing for a sibling-like relationship. The principle also applies to persons of the same sex who then become brothers or sisters and are expected to treat each other as real siblings would.

3 This mode of thought is vividly described by others such as Goodenough (1949) and Gladwin and Sarason (1953) for Chuuk. Goodenough (1949, p. 618) writes: 'The young man must be constantly on the alert so as not to miss the rare opportunities which come his way to arrange a rendezvous.'

4 In the past, this could mean breaking the little toe of the girl or woman or leaving scars (*nekinek*) on the body, ideally in an area such as between the upper inner thighs. Upon encountering this mark, the next man to engage in a sexual relationship with the woman would discover that he had been defeated in the race to do so.

5 The names used here and below are pseudonyms. Certain explicit interview content has been omitted to protect the identity of the interviewees.

## References

Caughey, J.L., 1977. *Fáánakkar: Cultural values in a Micronesian society*. University of Pennsylvania Publications in Anthropology no. 2. Philadelphia: Department of Anthropology, University of Pennsylvania.

Dernbach, C.B., 2005. Popular religion: A cultural and historical study of Catholicism and spirit possession in Chuuk, Micronesia. PhD thesis, University of Iowa.

FSM Department of Health and Social Affairs, 2014. *Federated States of Micronesia family health and safety study: A prevalence study on violence against women*. FSM Department of Health and Social Affairs.

Gladwin, T., 1953. The role of man and woman on Truk: A problem of personality and culture. *Transactions of the New York Academy of Sciences*, Series II 15 (8), 305–309.

Gladwin, T. and Sarason, S.B., 1953. *Truk: Man in paradise*. New York: Wenner-Gren Foundation for Anthropological Research.

Goodenough, W.H., 1949. Premarital freedom on Truk: Theory and practice. *American Anthropologist*, 51, 615–620.

Goodenough, W.H., 1951. *Property kin and Community on Truk*. Yale University Publications in Anthropology no. 46. New Haven, CN: Department of Anthropology, Yale University. Reprinted 1978. Hamden, CN: Archon Books.

Goodenough, W.H., 2002. *Under heavens brow: Pre-Christian religious tradition in Chuuk*. Memoirs of the American Philosophical Society, 246. Philadelphia, PA: The American Philosophical Society.

Hambruch, P. and Eilers, A., 1936. Ponape 2. Teilband. In: G. Thinenius (ed), *Ergebnisse der Südsee-Expedition*. Hamburg: Friedrichsen, De Gruyter, 1908–1910.

Hanlon, D., 1988. *Upon a stone altar: A history of the island of Pohnpei to 1890*. Honolulu: University of Hawai'i Press.

Hezel, F.X., 1984. Cultural patterns in Trukese suicide. *Ethnology*, 23, 193–206.

Hezel, F.X., 1989. Suicide and the Micronesian family. *The Contemporary Pacific*, 1 (1), 43–74.

Hezel, F., 1999. American Anthropology's contribution to social problems research in Micronesia. In: R. Kiste and M. Marshall (eds), *American Anthropology in Micronesia*. Honolulu: University of Hawaii Press, 301–325.

Hezel, F.X., 2001. *The new shape of old island cultures: A half century of social change in Micronesia*. Honolulu: University of Hawai'i Press.

Hezel, F.X., 2013. *Making sense of Micronesia: The logic of Pacific Island culture*. Honolulu: University of Hawai'i Press.

Larson, B., 1989. Sojourning and personhood: College students return to Truk, Federated States of Micronesia. PhD thesis, University of Hawaii.

Marshall, M., 1977. The nature of nurture. *American Ethnologist*, 4 (4), 643–662.

Marshall, M., 1979. *Weekend warriors: Alcohol in a Micronesian culture*. Mountain View, CA: Mayfield.

Marshall, M., 1983 [1981]. Sibling sets as building blocks in Greater Trukese society. In: M. Marshall (ed), *Siblingship in Oceania: Studies in the meaning of kin relations*, 201–224. Lanham: University Press of America.

Marshall, M., 2004. *Namoluk beyond the reef: The transformation of a Micronesian community*. Boulder, CO: Westview.

Moral, B., 1996. Conceptualisation de la mujer, del cuerpo de la sexualidad en Chuuk, Micronesia. Donostia: PhD thesis, Universidad del Pais Vasco/Euscal Herriko Unibertsitatea.

Moral, B., 1998. The Chuukese women's status. Traditional and modern elements. In: V. Keck (ed), *Common worlds and single lives: Constituting knowledge in Pacific societies*. Oxford: Berg, 274–284.

Moral Ledesma, B., 2000. Sexe des femmes, sexe des soeurs. Les organes génitaux féminins à Chuuk (Micronésie). *Journal de la Société des Océanistes*, 110 (2), 49–63.

Petersen, G., 2009. *Traditional Micronesian societies: Adaption, integration, and political organization*. Honolulu: University of Hawaii Press.

Rauchholz, M., 2008. Demythologizing adoption: From the practice to the effects of adoption in Chuuk, Micronesia. *Pacific Studies*, 31 (3/4), 156–181.

Rauchholz, M., 2010. Towards an understanding of adoption, person, and emotion: The ideal norm and reality of life amongst the Chuukese of Micronesia. PhD thesis, Ruprecht- Karls University Heidelberg.

Rauchholz, M., 2016. Masculine sexuality, violence and sexual exploitation in Micronesia. *The Asia Pacific Journal of Anthropology*, 17 (3–4), 342–358. doi:10.1080/14442213.2016.1196724

Schlesier, E., 1953. *Die Erscheinungsformen des Männerhauses und das Klubwesen in Mikronesien*. Eine ethno-soziologische Untersuchung. 'S-Gravenhage: Mouton.

Smith, S., 2014. The reproductive lives of Chuukese women: Transnationalism in Guam and Chuuk. PhD thesis, University of South Florida.

Smith, S., 2019. Gender, relationships and sexual violence in the lives of women from Chuuk, Micronesia. *Journal of Aggression, Maltreatment and Trauma*, 28 (2), 145–165. doi:10.1080/10926771.2018.1494236

Swartz, M.J., 1958. Sexuality and aggression on Romonum, Truk. *American Anthropologist*, 60 (3), 467–486.

# 15 Gender inequality and Pacific-led solutions for a global problem

*Fiona Hukula*

> … we're at a critical point in Pacific history. Greater levels of political commitment are required to ensure that our collective efforts are gender responsive on all fronts. Gender equality and empowerment must be at the core of our regional and national planning actions, policy development and funding allocations.
>
> Stuart Michin, Director General, Secretriate Pacific Community (SPC) (SPC 2021a)

## Introduction

The Blue Pacific Continent is known for its vast ocean, its unique cultures and its diversity. The majority of families and communities across our small islands rely on tourism, fisheries and agriculture as primary sources of income. Within this idyllic island setting, issues of sex and gender are paramount. As well as providing a cultural reference point for gender diversity (see, e.g., Veukiso-Ulugia et al. Chapter 3; Futter-Puati Chapter 4) the region is also marked by serious gender inequity. Gender inequity is evident in homes, across communities and in political leadership. Its most damaging form is the ongoing violence perpetrated against our women and girls.

To address gender inequality in the region, we need to address inequity across several fronts all at the same time, and one of these, and the focus my much of my work, is ending violence against women and girls. The effects of violence against women and girls affect their safety and ability to complete their education, generate an income, fulfil their hopes and dreams and take on leadership roles meaningfully and fully. Countries, including the men and boys in them, cannot prosper when half the population remains under the threat of violence.

One of our countries in our region, the one in which I was born, is ranked 161 out of 162, just ahead of Yemen, in the United National Gender Inequality Index (UNDP n.d.). Motivated personally and professionally to address the lack of women's representation in parliament and to end violence against women and girls, in this chapter I provide an overview of our regional political commitments to addressing gender inequality and the role of donor sponsored

DOI: 10.4324/9781003142072-18

programmes to meet these goals. Following this, I offer some local Pacific-led solutions to addressing violence against women and girls followed by my concerns about the effect the COVID-19 pandemic has had on these successes and what this means for ongoing success.

### *Women and political leadership*

Women's political leadership in the Pacific is amongst the lowest in the world. There is also a lack of women's leadership in senior managerial and administrative roles in Pacific governments and State-owned enterprises. While the private sector has been more progressive in supporting women's leadership, it remains evident that this leadership is lacking across the Pacific region. The Blue Pacific has some of the poorest rates of women's participation and representation in parliament, with some countries not having any women representatives at all. At the time of writing, Vanuatu has just elected its first female MP, and after having no elected women leaders in the last term of government (2017–2022), only two were elected in this recent, violent election in Papua New Guinea. Decision-makers at the highest level of government in Papua New Guinea level perpetuate this inequality by failing to safeguard seats for women. In contrast, the Autonomous Region of Bougainville, reserves three seats for women leaders in its assembly. The fact that this most recent election was so violent and destructive, crippled with bribery, shows just how unsafe standing for election is for women in Papua New Guinea, but we need more women leaders for the country to progress.

Only two women have ever been head of state in a Pacific country – President Hilda Heine, Republic of Marshall Islands (2016–2020) and Prime Minister Hon. Fiame Mataafa, Samoa (2022—). Having women in Parliament is important for diversity of thinking and experience but it can also be a way to ensure that women's leadership moves beyond the confines of home, church and the local community. Inequity in leadership at a high level is but one of the many measures one can use to assess gender inequality in our region. Another reason for needing and wanting women in parliament where key decisions and policies are made is to bring light to the even more urgent issue of gender-based violence, a significant development issue that is a concern for all of us and to which our response will determine our progress into the future.

### *Violence against women and girls: what the numbers say*

Across the Blue Pacific, significant resources have been put into Family Health and Safety Studies (Kiribati, Solomon Islands, Samoa) and Demographic Health surveys (Papua New Guinea), as well as other research to assess gender inequality and the prevalence of gender-based violence. Sadly, the resounding message from these studies tell us that the Pacific is a seriously unsafe space for women and girls. In Kiribati, the Family Health and Support study (SPC 2010) found that 68% of ever-partnered women aged 15–49 had ever experienced violence. In the Solomon Islands, the Health and Safety study (SPC 2009) found that 64% of ever-partnered women aged 15–49 reported having experienced physical or sexual violence, or both, by an intimate partner and 42% of women reported experiencing physical and/or sexual partner violence in the last 12 months. The National Inquiry into Family Violence in Samoa (Samoa Office of the Ombudsman/NHRI Samoa 2018) found that family violence affects almost all families, with 60% of women experiencing intimate partner violence in their lifetime. In Papua New Guinea, the Demographic Health Survey 2016–2018 (NSO and ICF 2019) reports that 63% of ever-married women who were interviewed had experienced physical, sexual or emotional violence at the hands of an intimate partner, with physical violence the most common type of violence (54%) followed by emotional violence (51%). And violence against our trans women sisters is also concerning (see, e.g., Boli-Neo et al., Chapter 12). While one powerful image of the Blue Pacific Continent portrays it as an idyllic island region, each of these surveys, as well as others, repeatedly show that as women we endure levels of endemic proportions, and at rates far higher than the already high global average of 35% (Pacific Women 2022). Sadly, for our daughters and granddaughters (sons and grandsons), the rates of sexual abuse against children, and incest are also disturbing, not only in Palau (Kuartei 2005) and Pitcairn (Oliver 2009) but elsewhere.[1]

## Gender equality frameworks and commitments in the Blue Pacific

Pacific nations have made significant commitments to ending gender inequality. In 1994, the Pacific came together as a region to adopt a regional framework for the promotion of gender equity — the Pacific Platform for Action on the Advancement of Women and Gender Equality, known locally as the PPA. Concerned by the lack of progress seen in our communities following this commitment, Pacific leaders of the region rallied again in 2012 at the 43rd Pacific Islands Forum in Rarotonga, Cook Islands, to announce the Pacific Leaders Gender Equality Declaration to bring about much-needed gender equality (Pacific Islands Forum 2012). This declaration bought renewed focus, commitment and energy to lifting the status of women in the Pacific and empowering them to be active participants in economic, political and social life and thereby ending gender inequality. Specifically, the declaration focused on six key areas:

1. Gender responsive government programmes and policies
2. Decision making
3. Economic empowerment
4. Ending violence against women
5. Health
6. Education

Since 2012, annual assessments relevant to the declaration have been undertaken. Progress in bringing about tangible action set forth by this declaration was initially slow, however, in 2014 and 2015 it was acknowledged that progress had been made in the following areas:

> electoral reform, legislative reform for gender based violence, improved support services for the victims of violence, the implementation of projects to promote economic empowerment and sustainable livelihoods, improved access to reproductive health services and a groundswell of activity around strengthening the capacity of women as potential leaders.
>
> (PIFS 2016, p. 7)

In the 2016 assessment of the declaration, it was also reported that there had been, 'an increase in women reporting on domestic violence, accessing counselling services, receiving government scholarships and senior level appointments to the public sector' (PIFS 2016, p. 7).

The Biennial Pacific Development Reports produced by the Pacific Islands Forum Secretariat (2020) provide one of the most comprehensive ongoing assessments of gender equality in our region. This Biennial report measured progress on gender and was presented to the UN Secretary-General as the Pacific's single regional report on progress in the Pacific under the 2030 Agenda and the SIDS Accelerated Modalities for Action (SAMOA) Pathway. According to the 2020 Biennial Report, the Pacific has made significant progress towards addressing gender equality; however, efforts have been (and continue to be) hampered by harmful and discriminatory practices. The Biennial report identified numerous areas in need of improvement. One such area is the need to urgently and systematically integrate gender into legal and policy frameworks. The report also noted that the region has not adequately resourced the integration of gender equality priorities. This lack of resourcing of gender integration priorities means that the pursuit of gender equality remains a commitment but lacks support to turn it into action and produce the results we need.

In 2021, the Pacific Islands Forum Secretariat commissioned a review of the Pacific Leaders Gender Equality Declaration to determine the effectiveness and relevance of the Declaration as well as to gauge views from member countries and relevant partners on ways to better coordinate regional gender commitments. The review found that while the Declaration remained relevant for the region, there was a lack of ownership and visibility of the Declaration among all stakeholders.

Informed by the assessments made in relation to the Pacific Leaders Gender Equality Declaration as well as the 2030 Agenda for Sustainable Development Goals, the region developed an updated framework for achieving gender equity in the form of the Platform for Action on Gender Equality and Women's Human Rights 2018–2030 (Pacific Community 2018). The Pacific Platform provides a roadmap for achieving gender equality and enhancing the well-being of all women and girls. By reference to women and girls, it directs attention to all women and girls, not just some. This means young women, older women, rural women, women with disabilities, women with diverse sexual orientations and gender identities, and Indigenous women. The inclusion of Indigenous women is important in colonised countries and territories, including New Caledonia, American Samoa, and the Federated States of Micronesia, as well as in Fiji, where British colonial practices of bringing indentured labour from India to Fiji caused the Indigenous iTaukei people to be marginalised, contributing to ongoing political and other tensions.

The Pacific Platform for Action was designed to support the implementation of commitments made in other global, regional and national instruments, and more specifically through the Pacific Leaders Gender Equality Declaration and Sustainable Development Goal 5 – Achieve gender equality and empower all women and girls. It serves as a tool for accelerating the implementation of the Pacific Leaders Gender Equality Declaration. While this is a regional plan, it provides the framework for local responses. And there are some truly remarkable local responses being designed, implemented and evaluated across our sea of islands, as I will highlight later in this chapter.

To progress these commitments, Leaders have committed to implement specific national policy actions to progress gender equality, and each of these regional policy frameworks provides a locally relevant framework to advancing gender equality in the region. These regional frameworks are critical to the localisation of global frameworks and commitments in our own settings. Importantly they provide the Blue Pacific with collective priorities relating to advancing gender equality. National policies to address and mainstream gender are also evident in a number of Pacific countries and most also have gender-related policies that include the needs of persons with disabilities; Vanuatu is the most recent Pacific county to launch a National Gender Equality Policy (Government of the Republic of Vanuatu 2021).

In addition to these regional frameworks, the governments of the Blue Pacific have ratified a number of international Conventions, as per the UN Treaty Body Database (see https://tbinternet.ohchr.org/SitePages/Home.aspx). All Pacific Island nations have ratified the Convention on the Rights of the Child. Excluding Tonga and Palau, all other Pacific Island nations have ratified the Convention on the Elimination of all forms of Discrimination Against Women. Niue and Tokelau ratified Convention through the Government of New Zealand.

There are numerous areas where a global commitment has translated into local action. Under the pioneering leadership of former member of parliament and Minister for Community Development, Dame Carol Kidu, the *Lukautim Pikinini Act* (Child Welfare Act) was passed into law in Papua New Guinea in response to the country's commitment to the Convention of the Rights of the Child. While the original law did not change the minimum age of marriage for young women, a subsequent revision in 2015 increased the minimum age from 16 to 18 years, bringing the country's law into line with the Convention on the Rights of the Child (Library of Congress 2016).

Although most Pacific Governments have ratified the Convention on the Elimination of all forms of Discrimination Against Women, there are still gaps in implementation and action. One of the key challenges to acting on the articles in this Convention and the Convention on the Rights of the Child is the lack of resources and capacity to operationalise and implement policy. Donor and development support remains key (at least for now) to the success of Blue Pacific actions towards bringing about gender equity.

Being a signatory to international conventions and being committed to changes in legislation does not necessarily translate to tangible protection for women and girls, or at least it takes time for the two to converge, as the above examples highlight. At other times our region has been ahead of global commitments, as was seen most recently in the collective call for urgent action on climate change, with Vanuatu seeking an opinion from the International Court of Justice on rights for the protection of nation-states from climate change.

## Regional initiatives: Donor and development support

For many years, donor and development partners have supported the work of civil society and governments to address gender inequality and gender issues are addressed in the implementation of their activities. Since 2012, the biggest donor investment in the region has been by the Australian Government through the Pacific Women Shaping Pacific Development initiative. This took the form of an AUD20 million investment over 10 years in 14 Pacific Islands Forum countries. The focus was on supporting women's leadership, economic empowerment, ending violence against women and girls, and enhancing women's agency. The programme ended in 2021 but was followed by a five-year AUD170 million Pacific Women Lead programme to be delivered through the Pacific Community. This new programme seeks to promote women's leadership and women's rights, and increase the effectiveness of regional gender equality efforts.

Also promoting gender equality is the European Union-funded Pacific Partnership on Ending Violence against Women and Girls. This five-year programme which began in 2018 is also supported by the governments of Australia and New Zealand and enables the Pacific Island Forum Secretariat, the Pacific Community and UN Women Pacific to work jointly under a common framework to address gender equality and end violence against women and girls. Each partner is responsible for one intervention area as defined by three programme outcomes:

- Outcome 1. Secretariat of the Pacific Community (SPC): Enhance Pacific Youth's formal in-school and informal education about gender equality and prevention of violence against women and girls. This is important for achieving transformational change.
- Outcome 2. UN Women: Promote gender-equitable social norms at individual and community levels to prevent violence against women and girls and ensure survivors have access to quality response services.
- Outcome 3. The Pacific Islands Forum Secretariat (PIFS): Empower national and regional civil society organisations to advocate, monitor and report on regional and on government commitments to enhance gender equality and end violence against women and girls.

This five-year programme works in Pacific Island countries and territories to strengthen and support partnerships between governments and civil society to promote gender equality, prevent violence against women and girls and increase access to good quality services for the survivors of gender-based violence. The programme makes an important contribution to work on gender in the region since much of this work has been led by civil society and grassroots activism. It is important for national and regional civil society organisations to have the skills to advocate and monitor gender commitments in the region so as to actively participate in dialogue with governments. Engaging with a wide range of civil society organisations and faith-based organisations will enable conversations and advocacy to reach beyond traditional activist groups. Involving men and boys as well as young people generally is key in this respect.

These donor and development funded and/or led initiatives are filling the gap in providing resources that our national and local level governments often lack. While they provide technical support to address gender inequality in the region, it is also important to measure the outcomes and progress of these programmes using a Pacific-informed lens that takes into consideration the lived experience and challenges of addressing gender equality in the Pacific.

## Pacific-led solutions to addressing violence against women and girls

Across the Pacific are numerous homegrown initiatives to address violence against women and girls that have developed into networks and movements of women and women activists within countries and between them. These efforts have a long history, with Pacific feminists and women's rights activists, most notably in Fiji, leading the way in advocating for the rights of women and girls in all of their diversity and providing services to support and complement government provision.

Fiji has been a pioneer and beacon of light in the region and has played a key role in mentoring and supporting regional initiatives. Led by a group of feminist activists, Fiji established the Fiji Women's Crises Centre in 1984, the first Centre of its kind in the Pacific to support survivors of gender-based violence.[2] It now has several branches across the country and has provided services to thousands of women since it opened (Fiji Women's Crisis Centre 2022a). The Centre has also been involved in various high-level advocacy campaigns and initiatives both in Fiji and within the region. One example of their regional influence can be seen in the first Pacific Regional Workshop on Violence Against Women and the setting up of the Pacific Women's Network Against Violence Against Women in 1992. Building on the success and learning from the Fiji Women's Crisis Centre, similar centres have been established in Vanuatu (1992) and Tonga (where it has taken the name Women and Children's Crisis Centre, 2009). Both centres have been instrumental in leading advocacy, engaging in research and supporting the survivors of gender-based violence. In Tonga, a local radio programme, *Fanguna*, was broadcast to increase awareness and reduce violence, and crisis housing is provided by the *Mo'ui Fiefia Safe Hous*. In total 12 Pacific countries, including Cook Islands, Federated States of Micronesia, Fiji, Kiribati. Nauru, Papua New Guinea, Marshall Islands, Samoa, Tonga, Tuvalu and Vanuatu (see https://pacificwomen.org/crisis-centres/) have dedicated support services for survivors of domestic violence.

There are some promising examples of gender-based violence referral pathways being adopted in the Pacific. SafeNet is an initiative from the United Nations Joint Global Programme on Essential Services for Women and Girls Subject to Violence being piloted worldwide, including in the Pacific region in the Solomon Islands and Kiribati (SPC 2021b). The SafeNet referral system is a network of government, non-government and frontline service providers for survivors of sexual and gender-based violence and enables women to access support and assistance in a timely way. After several years of development by SafeNet members, and with the support of the UN Women Fiji multi-country office, the Solomon Islands SafeNet guidebook was published in 2019. The SafeNet Initiative is also being implemented in Kiribati. Pacific knowledge exchange is also occurring, with SafeNet study tours with delegates from the Federated States of Micronesia and Kiribati visiting the Solomon Islands in 2020–2021. The continued support and mentorship of the Fiji Women's Crises Centre to civil society networks in Pacific Island countries also provide the impetus for partnership and exchange. These initiatives of learning and exchange enable Pacific people to share best practices, network and form alliances for better advocacy and regional engagement. Cross-Pacific interaction is particularly important during this time of climate crisis, COVID-19 and intensified geopolitical interest in the region.

Another important example of a locally led initiative is provided by the Highlands Human Rights Defenders in Papua New Guinea. The Human Rights Defenders network, as they are commonly referred to, is a network of women who advocate for, respond to, and work towards the prevention of violence against women and girls. Their actions include addressing gender-based violence linked to the disturbing sorcery accusations that are plaguing the country. Initially formed as an alliance of women from tribal groups in conflict to address tribal violence in parts of the Highlands, the Highlands Human Rights Defenders network brings together local civil society organisations such as Kup Women for Peace and Kafe Urban Women's Association. These groups have now taken on a broader role of advocacy and are first responders to women, children and communities who face various forms of gender-based violence, including sorcery accusation-related violence. Supported by Oxfam, this network of women now links to other human rights defenders in other parts of Papua New Guinea.

Churches have an important role to play in the daily lives of most Pacific Islanders. It is no surprise then that they have a key role to play in advancing gender equality, including addressing violence against women and girls (see, e.g., Sharma 2014; Gibbs 2016). In Fiji, the Anglican Church has established the House of Sarah to provide a safe haven for those who are vulnerable to abuse. Supported by UN Women, House of Sarah provides counselling support, undertakes advocacy with church leaders on gender-based violence, and supports regional exchanges between the Anglican Church in Solomon Islands, Vanuatu, Papua New Guinea and the Diocese of Polynesia. In Papua New Guinea, the Catholic Church has been instrumental in addressing violence against women and girls in a variety of ways, including working with men. Father Phil Gibbs and Caritas have been pioneers in this space, training male advocates, as has Sr Lorraine Garasu of the Nazarene Rehabilitation Centre in the Autonomous Region of Bougainville. Plagued with the trauma of a violent decade-long civil war, the Nazareth Rehabilitation Centre has engaged men and boys in a variety of programmes to change gender norms and end violence against women and girls. These programmes have included Healing of Memory Workshops as well as *Planim Save Kamap Strongpela*, a joint UN Women project that involved men and boys as well as women and girls.

In addition to these locally led programmes and a growing body of academic and other work, as Pacific Islanders, we are storytellers and as such, our region has produced much advocacy material through TV series, film, photo voice and digital storytelling to advocate for and create conversations about gender equality and ending violence against women and girls. The number of arts-based approaches contributing to these conversations is growing each year. *Love Patrol* (2007–2015), a ni-Vanuatu TV series which ran for eight years, was produced by Wan Smolbag and has been viewed across the Pacific. While funded to address HIV, it also addressed issues of gender inequality and violence, family life and sexual relationships, as well as sexuality and gender diversity. A Pacific Community Filming Consortium has recently been established and has initiated a Film4gender Project. Numerous films have been produced that address issues of gender inequality, particularly as it relates to violence. *Hero-ine* (2020) focuses on a female character trying to access police and justice services following an incident of gender-based violence, and addresses the bias by male police and others in women's access to such services. *Te Ala kite Mae* (A Path Towards Violence) (2020) examines the impact of gender-based violence, and alcohol, on a young Tuvaluan couple living in the village. Continuing to ensure women in all their diversity are included in art-based work, the film *Weaving the Streets* (2020) tells the story of a trans woman and her struggles moving from a village to the city as a sex worker, and her determination and courage to face violence and discrimination. Films that address sorcery accusation-related violence in PNG include those produced by *Yumi Sanap Strong* (2022).

## COVID-19: a risk to progress

Like elsewhere, gains relating to gender equality in our region have been threatened with the global COVID-19 pandemic. Lockdowns and restrictions means that formal employment has been affected, especially for those who work in the tourism and hospitality industry. Violence against women is reported to have increased in several countries of the region. It has also become harder for women to seek assistance due to lockdowns. Lockdowns have also affected women's ability to access sexual and reproductive health services. Care of the most vulnerable members of community such as persons with disabilities, the elderly and children have been left to women. In cases where women have been required to work from home, the balancing of domestic duties and work commitments has created an added responsibility for women.

One of the greatest concerns relating to COVID-19 has been the increase in gender-based violence. The toll-free national helpline in Fiji recorded a 300% increase in domestic violence-related calls one month after curfews and lockdowns were implemented (Young 2021). Compared to 87 and 187 calls in February and March 2020 respectively, in April 2020 there were 527 recorded calls to the helpline in Fiji (UN Women 2020). Similarly, Tonga reported a 54% increase in calls for help (UN Women 2020). In Samoa, during the first six weeks of lockdown, the Samoa Victim Support Group responded to 150 more calls than usual through the helpline (UN Women 2020), with 46 distress calls resulting in police intervention to address domestic violence in the home (Lesa and Apelu 2020). In Papua New Guinea, the 1 Talk Kaunselling helpline increased its call hours and capacity in anticipation of an increase in calls (Child Fund 2020). Women in the Pacific are always resilient and with COVID-19, and the lockdown, women and the civil societies that work to support them have had to be even more so.

Women's groups have linked the increase in domestic violence to the rise in unemployment and the financial difficulties which have resulted from the pandemic. While family violence or violence between intimate partners is the most common form of violence reported, other forms of gender-based violence such as rape and sexual harassment remain a serious cause for concern.

## Concluding remarks

In order to progress gender equality, it is essential to view gender as being about both men and women and appreciate the importance of leadership in supporting equality for all. It is crucial that Pacific women take leadership roles in all spheres of life and the lack of women's leadership at the highest political level contributes to slowing down progress. The importance of women's voices for diversity and inclusion cannot be understated, especially during these trying times.

While various commitments to gender equality have been made through the Pacific Leaders Gender Equality Declaration as well as the ratification of international instruments such as the Convention on the Elimination of all forms of Discrimination Against Women, much of the grass-roots action to address gender inequality in the Pacific has been supported by donors and development partners which affects the sustainability of such initiatives and the ability of governments to continue to support programmes.

Gender-based violence is one of, if not the most important obstacle to not only reducing inequality between men and women but also building sustainable, resilient communities. While violence against women is the most prevalent form of gender-based violence in our region, marginalised groups including persons with disabilities and sexuality and gender diverse people also suffer from violence. The trying times that we find ourselves in require us to rethink how we live in this world and there are some elements of our lives that require continued conversation – in edited books such as this, in policy spaces, in places of learning such as schools and universities, and within our homes and communities.

## Notes

1 Data on incest is difficult to determine. For media reports of cases in Papua New Guinea see, for example, Papua New Guinea Today (2015) and PNG Daily (2020).
2 For a history of the Fiji Women's Crisis Centre see Fiji Women's Crisis Centre 2022b and 2022c.

## References

Child Fund, 2020. Domestic violence helpline in Papua New Guinea to expand during COVID-19 pandemic. *ChildFund Australia*, 19 May. Available from: https://www.childfund.org.au/media-news/domestic-violence-helpline-in-papua-new-guinea-to-expand-during-covid-19-pandemic/ [Accessed 15 August 2022].

Fiji Women's Crisis Centre, 2022a. FWCC and branches total new cases seen. *Fiji Women's Crisis Centre*. Available from: http://www.fijiwomen.com/publications/statistics/fwcc-branches-total-statistics/ [Accessed 15 August 2022].

Fiji Women's Crisis Centre, 2022b. Our history. *Fiji Women's Crisis Centre*. Available from: https://www.fijiwomen.com/about/our-history/ [Accessed 15 August 2022].

Fiji Women's Crisis Centre, 2022c. Since 13th August 1984. 38 years on, we are more in numbers, stronger and still marching for women's human rights, democracy and rule of law. *Fiji Women's Crisis Centre* [Facebook], 12 August. Available from: https://www.facebook.com/FijiWomen/videos/since-13th-august-1984-38-years-on-we-are-more-in-numbers-stronger-and-still-mar/3619999127912691/ [Accessed 15 August 2022].

Gibbs, P., 2016. Men's matters: Changing masculine identities in Papua New Guinea. In: A. Biersack, M. Jolly, and M. Macintyre (eds), *Gender violence and human rights: Seeking justice in Fiji, Papua New Guinea and Vanuatu*. Canberra: ANU Press, 127–158.

Government of the Republic of Vanuatu, 2021. *Government of the Republic of Vanuatu National Gender Equity Policy 2020-2030*. Port Vila: Government of the Republic of Vanuatu. Available from: https://www.sistalibrary.com.vu/wp-content/uploads/2021/11/NGEP-1.pdf [Accessed 15 August 2022].

Hero-ine, 2020. Film. Directed by Anouk Ride. Solomon Islands: Sukwadi Media.

Kuartei, S., 2005. Incest in Palau: 'Delemumuu undressed.' *Pacific Health Dialog*, 12 (1), 84–91.

Lesa, L. and Apelu, L., 2020. Help is not on lockdown: Samoan shelters and helplines continue operating through the pandemic. *Spotlight Initiative*, 21 September. Available from: https://www.spotlightinitiative.org/fr/node/36175 [Accessed 15 August 2022].

Library of Congress, 2016. *Papua New Guinea: Changes to marriage laws to be introduced. Library of Congress*, 23 August. Available from: https://www.loc.gov/item/global-legal-monitor/2016-08-23/papua-new-guinea-changes-to-marriage-laws-to-be-introduced/ [Accessed 15 August 2022].

Love Patrol, 2007–2015. TV. Vanuatu: Wan Smolbag Theatre.

NSO and ICF, 2019. *Papua New Guinea demographic and health survey 2016-18*. Port Moresby, Papua New Guinea. Available from: https://dhsprogram.com/publications/publication-fr364-dhs-final-reports.cfm [Accessed 15 August 2022].

Oliver, D., 2009. *Justice, legality and the rule of law: Lessons from the Pitcairn prosecutions*. New York: Oxford University Press.

Pacific Community, 2018. Pacific platform for action on gender equality and women's human rights 2018–2030, part 1. Available from: https://www.sistalibrary.com.vu/wp-content/uploads/2020/05/Pacific_Platform_for_Action_on_Gender_Equality_Part1_EN.pdf [Accessed 15 August 2022].

Pacific Islands Forum, 2012. *Pacific leaders gender equality declaration, 30 August 2012, Rarotonga, Cook Islands*. Available from: https://www.forumsec.org/2012/08/30/plged/ [Accessed 15 August 2022].

Pacific Islands Forum Secretariat (PIFS), 2016. *Pacific Leaders gender equality declaration trend assessment report 2012–2016*. Available from: https://www.aidsdatahub.org/sites/default/files/resource/pacific-leaders-gender-equality-declaration-2016.pdf [Accessed 15 August 2022].

Pacific Islands Forum Secretariat, 2020. *The 2020 Biennial Pacific Sustainable Development Report*. Available from: https://www.forumsec.org/wp-content/uploads/2021/03/Biennial-Pacific-Sustainable-Development-Report_12112020_FINAL.pdf [Accessed 24 August 2022].

Pacific Women, 2022. *Ending violence against women* [online]. Available from: https://pacificwomen.org/our-work/focus-areas/ending-violence-against-women/ [Accessed 24 August 2022].

Papua New Guinea Today, 2015. Incest cases in PNG's East New Britain Province still high. *Papua New Guinea Today*, 22 February. Available from: https://news.pngfacts.com/2015/02/incest-cases-in-pngs-east-new-britain.html [Accessed 15 August 2022].

PNG Daily, 2020. *Kokopo police charge man for incest* [Facebook], 10 June. Available from: https://www.facebook.com/pngdaily/posts/kokopo-police-charge-man-for-incestby-the-post-courier-10-june-2020a-50-year-old/257705998989721/ [Accessed 15 August 2020].

Samoa Office of the Ombudsman/NHRI Samoa, 2018. *National Public Inquiry into family violence*. Available from: https://ombudsman.gov.ws/wp-content/uploads/2018/09/National-Inquiry-Report-into-Family-Violence_-State-of-Human-Rights-Report-2018-English.pdf [Accessed 15 August 2022].

Secretariat of the Pacific Community (SPC), 2009. *Solomon Islands family health and safety study: A study on violence against women and children*. Noumea, New Caledonia: Secretariat of the Pacific Community. Available from: https://pacific.unfpa.org/sites/default/files/pub-pdf/SolomonIslandsFamilyHealthandSafetyStudy.pdf [Accessed 15 August 2022].

Secretariat of the Pacific Community (SPC), 2010. *Kiribati family health and support study: A study on violence against women and children*. Noumea, New Caledonia: Secretariat of the Pacific Community. Available from: https://pacific.unfpa.org/sites/default/files/pub-pdf/Kiribati-Family-Health-and-Support-Study_0.pdf [Accessed 15 August 2022].

Secretariat of the Pacific Community (SPC), 2021a. 14th Triennial Conference of Pacific Women opens with call for more inclusive development. *Pacific Community*, 28 April. Available from: https://www.spc.int/updates/blog/2021/04/14th-triennial-conference-of-pacific-women-opens-with-call-for-more-inclusive [Accessed 15 August 2022].

Secretariat of the Pacific Community (SPC), 2021b. 14th Triennial Conference discusses home-grown initiatives to counter gender based violence. *Pacific Community*, 29 July. Available from: https://hrsd.spc.int/node/838 [Accessed 15 August 2022].

Sharma, G., 2014. *Violent men: Perpetrators and forgotten victims - From abused boys to perpetrators of male violence – A pastoral theological strategy for prevention of male violence against women and children in Fiji*. Masters thesis. University of Auckland. Available from: https://researchspace.auckland.ac.nz/handle/2292/22423 [Accessed 15 August 2022].

Te Ala kite Mae, 2020. Film. Directed by Tala Simeti. Tuvalu.

UNDP, n.d. Gender inequality index (GII). *UNDP, Human Development Reports* [online]. Available from: https://hdr.undp.org/data-center/thematic-composite-indices/gender-inequality-index#/indicies/GII [Accessed 15 August 2022].

UN Women, 2020. Across the Pacific, crisis centres respond to COVID-19 amid natural disasters. *UN Women, Asia and the Pacific*, 11 June. Available from: https://asiapacific.unwomen.org/en/news-and-events/stories/2020/06/across-the-pacific-region-crisis-centres-respond-to-increased-cases-of-violence [Accessed 15 August 2022].

Weaving the Streets, 2020. Film. Directed by Larry Thomas and Joji Nabalarua. Fiji: X'isle Productions.

Young, M., 2021. A Pacific regional approach to implementing domestic violence legislation. *Secretariat of the Pacific Community*, 23 August. Available from: https://www.spc.int/updates/blog/blog/2021/08/a-pacific-regional-approach-to-implementing-domestic-violence-legislation [Accessed 15 August 2022].

Yumi Sanap Strong. 2022. Yumi Sanap Strong. [Facebook]. Available from: https://www.facebook.com/yumisanapstrong [Accessed 15 August 2022].

# Index

Note: *Italicized*, **bold** and ***bold italics*** refer to figures, tables and boxes. Page numbers followed by "n" refer to notes.